THE BACK PAIN SOURCEBOOK

The
Back Pain
Sourcebook

SECOND EDITION

BY
STEPHANIE LEVIN-GERVASI
FOREWORD BY JAMES F. ZUCHERMAN, M.D.

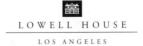

LOWELL HOUSE

LOS ANGELES

NTC/Contemporary Publishing Group

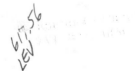

Library of Congress Cataloging-in-Publication Data

Levin-Gervasi, Stephanie.
      The back pain sourcebook: everything you need to know / by Stephanie Levin-Gervasi.
         p.   cm.
      Includes bibliographical references and index.
      ISBN 0-7373-0015-9
      1. Backache—Popular works. 2. Back—Care and hygiene.
      I. Title.
      RD771.B217L48   1995
      617.5'64—dc20   95-14200

Published by Lowell House, a division of NTC/Contemporary Publishing Group, Inc.
4255 West Touhy Avenue, Lincolnwood, Illinois 60646-1975 U.S.A.

Text design: Brenda Leach

Printed and bound in the United States of America
International Standard Book Number: 0-7373-0015-9
10 9 8 7 6 5 4 3 2 1

To the memory of my dear friend Jeremy Lustig,
whose courage and conviction taught me to never avert my eyes from the truth.

———————————————

Contents

FOREWORD

Back pain and its treatment is a complicated field, and an honest and comprehensive book that is useful to most back sufferers is a daunting task. As you will read, there is nothing more common than back pain in humans. Unfortunately, we, the potential and current victims, do not understand the disease process. This is a tragedy, since it is such a common ailment and mostly preventable. The author has adroitly gathered together the facts that we do have and the treatments that have proven themselves in terms of availability and effectiveness. There is a useful mix of anecdotal and objective factual material to make the book readable and practical. Anyone with first- or secondhand experience with spinal problems will find this comprehensive sourcebook fascinating as well as full of vital "what you can do" information.

In order to put this topic in perspective and understand why there are so many types of treatment to choose from, one has to appreciate the nature of painful spinal disease. Most episodes of spinal pain will resolve, no matter what is done, within six to twelve weeks of symptom onset. So whether you see your chiropractor, your general practitioner, your Feldenkrais practitioner, your acupuncturist, or your neighbor, chances are you're going to get well within a couple of months. This makes all of us back-health-care practitioners look good if we see patients soon enough after symptoms start.

Well-meaning expectations of healers are powerful. We all want our treatments to work, and we want to take credit for them when they do seem to work. So it's not surprising that once we believe that our treatment works, we selectively remember the facts that support that and tend to forget the instances when the treatment failed. Thus, we remain convinced that we are effective. With most of the patients responding so well early on in the clinical course of back disease, regardless of treatment, you can see how all the back-care practitioners feel that their type of treatment is usually successful. How many of our treatments for back pain appear to work because of our own and our patients' perceptual biases?

Understandably, the so-called placebo response, a normal human reaction, has powerful effects on a sufferer's symptoms. Medication has up to a 40-percent placebo response rate, meaning that four out of ten people who take a pill for a symptom will have improvement in the symptom even when the pill has nothing in it but sugar. The decision to go to a professional and get your back treated involves expectations and changes in your thinking and life patterns that may tend to induce an apparent healing, no matter what happens! Undergoing a frightening and painful procedure may carry a 60-percent placebo reaction rate.

Ultimately, the common denominator is pain. But pain is poorly understood and an unwieldy topic. One person's intolerable agony is another's mild discomfort. Sorting out objectively, then, which treatments are really most effective in relieving pain becomes complicated.

Doesn't medical research give us answers? Yes and no. Many aspects of disease are better understood than ever before. In fact, the last decade has seen a revolution in understanding the nature of back pain and how best to treat it. But there is still much more to learn, such as which physical therapy, chiropractic treatment, osteopathic manipulations, medication or spinal injections, and so on are most effective for a particular set of symptoms at a particular time.

We don't know specifically why the spinal tissue deteriorates with age, why some people have severe pain with a minor structural aberration and why another with severe abnormalities of the spinal structure may not have much in the way of symptoms. We can't tell with great accuracy in some situations whether surgery would be helpful or not. We don't have good ways to completely control chronic long-term pain, although we can make it better. The list continues, but every year significant pieces to the puzzle keep appearing, thanks to the very active research teams across the country.

During thirteen years on the staff at St. Mary's Spine Center and more recent seven years as the medical director of the St. Mary's Spine Center in San Francisco, we have had whirlwinds of change in management and understanding of back care. Originally, with Dr. Arthur White, the standard treatment for back and leg pain changed from bed rest and traction to dynamic stabilization training on an outpatient basis, thus allowing patients to remain as active as possible while keeping the back at rest.

Physical therapy segued from passive treatment with hot packs and ultrasound to educational "back" school and body-mechanic training, progressing individuals to their own independent gym or home exercise programs. The psychology of complex back problems was given its due attention, and specialists in chronic pain were recruited. Osteopathic physicians brought their manual skills to the treatment armamentarium. The therapeutic and diagnostic usefulness of fluoroscopically controlled spinal injects, established first at the St. Mary's Spine Center, soon made St. Mary's the foremost effective multidisciplinary spine center in the country. My staff and I developed improved instrumentation techniques for fusion to increase the success rate in those operations. Most recently, we developed the first laparascopic instrumented fusion technique, which is now in FDA clinical trials.

On the horizon we have artificial disks, bone morphogenic protein, cartilage transplantation, and the expanding knowledge base of the etiology of pain and how we may be able to control it. New surgical techniques are emerging, as is treatment of osteoporosis to slow the degenerative disease process in many elderly people.

Having stated the difficulties in finding the truth in the back-care field, the reader, with the solid, commonsense information this book provides, can make his or her own judgments and act accordingly. After all, as a spine physician and surgeon, my first and primary goal is to restore the perception of health and normalcy to individuals by the safest means available. I am ultimately most concerned with the outcome rather than the complex and subtle mechanism of a particular treatment. My own experience has borne out that many treatments work for many conditions as one single treatment seldom does. The job of the practitioner delivering spine care today is to remain as flexible and objective as possible in regard to treatment techniques. We must realize that no one particular treatment will appropriately serve all patients, and no individual practitioner can possess the skills to administer all treatments expertly. We must be triage experts so that referrals can enable levels of care to match the level of complexity of a particular problem and to assure that each treatment is most successful with a particular problem. Finally, as with other areas in health care, sorely little attention is given to prevention, which in my opinion could reduce the financial, psychological, and physical toll from back disease to a third of its present level.

—JAMES F. ZUCHERMAN, M.D.

ACKNOWLEDGMENTS

The fruition of this book would not have been possible without the help and encouragement of many. To everyone that gave generously of their time and expertise during the gathering of information and writing of *The Back Pain Sourcebook*, I am grateful. In particular, I would like to thank the following individuals for their valuable imput:

To the Medical Director of St. Mary's Spine Center, James F. Zucherman, M.D., for his extraordinary generosity, expert advice, and guidance whenever I knocked on his door for help. To Arthur H. White, M.D., medical director of Seton Spinecare for his time and generous library of information and insight into spine care. To Ron Friedman, M.D., for that one phone call. To Arthur Schuller, M.D., director of pain management at St. Mary's Spine Center for his sensitive and crucial insight on pain. To Richard Aptaker, D.O., chief of physical medicine and director of the spine clinic at Kaiser Permanente, San Franscisco for his time between patients to discuss back schools and spine exercises. To Kenneth Hsu, M.D., chief of orthopedics at St. Mary's Spine Center for the drawings in this book. To Mary Pullig Schatz, M.D., for her generous information on yoga and the back. To William C. Meeker, D.C, M.P.H., Dean of Research at Palmer College of Chiropractic-West for his time and willingness to educate me about chiropractics. To Paul Lipscomb, M.D., chief of orthopedics at Kaiser Permanente in Oakland for his time. To Karen Woodbury, D.C., for her immense help, encouragement, and work on my back. To Larry C. Forsberg for his help on acupuncture and herbs. To Pilates instructor Madelene Black, a heartful thanks for all your time and contacts. To Stephanie E. Clipper at the National Institute of Health for pertinent information at inception of this book. To Laura Hitchcock, Ph.D., and executive director of the National Chronic Pain Outreach Association for her insight and information. To Michael Castleman for his friendship and priceless direction. To Beverly Biondi, physical therapist, for her help on stabilization. To Linda Cogozzo at Rodmell Press for her encouragement. To Susan Branum, Joanne Lustig, Neal Powers, Peter de Zordo, Darcy Elman, Karen A. Perlroth, and the Center for Movement Education in San Francisco for their exquisite information on body work. To the National Cancer Institute for all their information. To the staff, particularly the volunteers, at Planetree Health Resource Center who gave of their time to help research my book. To my friend Susan Bistline for breakfast and inspiration on those difficult days. To each individual that gave of his or her time to educate me about their back problem. To my editor Bud Sperry for his encouragement and understanding my speed at the computer. And on the homefront, Luis and Camille.

INTRODUCTION

It's a medical nemesis and has been called the bane of the twentieth century. Victims spend a fortune going from practitioner to practitioner trying to cure it, and in the last twenty years an entire medical specialty has evolved to treat it.

Back pain is pervasive, striking men and women, the healthy and the unsuspecting. If you stand in a random crowd of twelve individuals, ten will bear one distinctive commonality: They suffer from back pain. Of the ten, half live with chronic problems, four tell you they've incurred debilitating life changes, and the other two have experienced at least two back attacks.

What's wrong with our backs? Is it our genes? Did our ancestors go to bed feeling great and wake up hunched over? Did they lean over to tie a shoe and then were unable to straighten up? Did your parents and grandparents bend over backward to do a good job only to be rewarded with back spasms? Did their backs, for no apparent reason, just slip out of place?

The back is a delicate mystery. Sure, our ancestors had their share of backaches, but by our current standards, it appears they managed either to live with it or control it. While some argue that our easy lifestyle is a detriment to our backbone, the statistics on back pain continue to rise. Back pain is a mind-boggling $50 billion problem that by all indications isn't going away.

On the hit list of ailments, back problems are surpassed only by the common cold. Eighty percent of the American population will be afflicted with back pain in their lifetime. If you've picked up this book, chances are you're already a statistic.

Oddly enough, the pervasiveness of backaches leads us to the conclusion that since such an overwhelming percentage of the population shares a back malady or two, our backs must be alike. Nothing could be further from the truth. Your back is as individual as your fingerprint. No two backs are alike, so what works for one back problem often does not work for another.

Confusion and understanding shroud back pain, which is not only continually perplexing but, like the weather, also highly unpredictable.

Many people never come to understand their back problems. When they encounter unpredictable pain, undetectable causes and apathetic specialists, suffering begins to pervade every crevice and corner of their lives.

But back pain does not have to be the end of the road. On the contrary, treating your back can be an opportunity for personal growth, a journey into self-discovery. I know, pain shouldn't have to be the segue into self-discovery; unfortunately, it often is.

For nearly twenty-five years I've suffered from chronic back pain. What precipitated the pages of this book was not a terrible accident or a debilitating spinal disability, but back pain in the prime of my life, followed by freedom from back pain for many years—and then a recurrence of that back pain again and again.

My first back event began atop a set of uneven parallel bars in a gymnastic tournament when I was in junior college in the late sixties. Straddling the high bar with my feet and hands, body taut to dismount backward, I slipped and, with a thud, landed on my back. Humiliated, I jumped up, assuring my horrified coach, who apologized profusely for not catching me, that everything was fine. Only my pride was hurt—or so I thought. A few days later my back was killing me. After a thorough examination and X rays, the doctor assured me nothing was wrong. But something was wrong. I became so terrified of falling on my back again that I quit gymnastics, turning away from a possible athletic scholarship to a large four-year university.

Athletic intent, however, coursed through my family's veins. I became a weekend terror on the ski slopes. I wasn't about to snowplow the bunny slopes while my friends braved the more advanced peaks. Without so much as a stretch, I went to the top. Oh, sure, I had my share of spills, skis flying in all directions, but luckily I only sprained a foot. I prided myself in knowing how to fall. Besides, at age twenty-four I was in great shape.

My thirst for competition required more than a weekend sport. Tennis was the rising star in Southern California. By my twenty-seventh birthday I was batting the tennis ball an average of two or three hours a day. Petite but feisty, I amazed my male opponents with a serve that sent their heads spinning. And I'll admit, a few times I returned from the courts to soak in a warm bath and put a hot pad on my back.

This should have been a warning, but who pays attention to a few creaky backbones and muscle spasms at twenty-seven? Besides, I figured I had discovered the key to the fountain of youth: Play hard, and change sports every few years.

A move to Europe put a damper on my tennis game. I didn't have the time, money, or inclination to spend an hour crossing a city to play. I returned to my childhood passion—dance. My passion on the dance floor made my sports enthusiasm look amateurish. I returned to the States to study. I studied modern dance and ballet, five days a week. I danced with an obsession few could understand. Ballet disciplined my entire life. My writing was better, my teaching easier, and I was happy. Unless, of course, my back acted up.

The classical ballerina stance is murder on a healthy back. It puts tremendous strain on the spine and neck. But I simply chalked up the strain to age. Never mind that I had a lithe spine and an arabesque to die for, a young ballerina I was not. While my mind didn't accept it, my body knew differently. At times the back pain was so intense that I actually missed class. During one painful bout I implored a friend to rush me to my chiropractor. I couldn't drive, because I couldn't move. The chiropractor put me on the table, rubbed heat on the affected area, positioned the table, and cracked my back. He suggested a respite from the dance floor.

I took a trip back to Europe—yes, with a backpack. For eight weeks I lugged clothes, guidebooks, and relics on my frail back. My back revolted and my neck tensed. To this day, I don't carry things on my back—not babies, books, or packs.

While in Europe I became interested in yoga, which is blissfully good for your body. Except that I dove into the gentle postures with the ferocity of a jockey intent on driving his slowish thoroughbred to the winner's circle. I wrenched my neck doing a headstand. Yoga is not a sport, nor is it about standing on your head simply because everyone else is doing it. For the first time since my fall from the uneven parallel bars, I began to think about my body. Were the back deities trying to tell me something? I stayed with yoga, becoming a kinder, gentler participant. I still practice yoga today. But I never stand on my head.

In 1983, at the age of thirty-four, I returned to Paris where the entire population complained of backaches. Funny, the guidebooks never mentioned this affliction, but in no time I understood why so many backs hurt. Besides lumpy mattresses left over from the Revolution, the kitchen sinks were built for midgets. Since everyone I knew had back problems, it was easy to find a *kinostheotique*—a cross between a chiropractor and an osteopath—whom I visited regularly to adjust my back and neck.

I continued to dance, fully aware that my back and neck were not happy campers. Then, horror of horrors, I broke my foot. No more dancing, no romantic walks through Paris, just five flights of stairs to tackle on crutches.

Five months later, I came back home and put my ballet slippers on for the last time. So concerned was I for my foot, I neglected to pay attention to the rest of my body. While warming up on the barre, I leaned into a classic arabesque position, and froze as a great pain ripped through my back. I couldn't move, and intuitively I knew my dancing career was facing its final curtain call.

By this time my chiropractor of twenty years had grown accustomed to my frantic calls begging for the laying on of hands. This time I got a lecture with the hands.

"I have no magic formula for your back, Stephanie. Think about a lifestyle change. Try walking, and then consider something kind for your body, like swimming." He added a few tidbits about the aging spine and muscle strain. A lifestyle change at my age? He had to be kidding.

I took up walking simply because anything else hurt too much. I wasn't ready for the pool. Once in a while I tried acupuncture, and I always appreciated a good massage. For the next few years, I would go for months pain free; then, mysteriously, my back would rage into spasm.

My husband and I moved to Northern California. Once, without thinking, I lifted a heavy box. Two days later I woke up riddled with neck and back pain. Lost without my old chiro standby, I thumbed through the phone directory and found a chiropractor. He wanted X rays and suggested treatment three times a week. Yipes, X rays, treatment three times a week, and my HMO didn't cover chiropractic care. I declined the weekly treatments but took the X ray. Unbeknownst to me, I was pregnant. Three weeks later I miscarried.

Loss builds reflection, and I began reading and re-evaluating my lifestyle. A year later I became pregnant again, and sailed through a glorious pregnancy without a pain in my back. Unfortunately, during my labor I suffered the most unimaginable back pain ever. I should have known that back pain at only two centimeter's dilation meant trouble. The doctor offered drugs, which I declined in my laborious state. I'll spare the details but simply state that nothing in the history of my back problems prepared me for sixteen hours of excruciating back labor, which thankfully resolved itself after the birth of my daughter.

Motherhood is wonderful, but it's very hard on the back. As a breast-feeding mom, I couldn't grasp the concept that I bring the baby to the breast, not the breast to the baby. For months my entire back, neck, and shoulders ached. The final straw that broke this back occurred nine months after my daughter's birth. I was in Las Vegas visiting family. An hour before flying home, I reached down to retrieve my daughter from the floor—and couldn't get up. My daughter perched on all fours, laughing, I, on all fours, was crying. The pain, homesteaded in my lower back, radiated throughout my body. Thank goodness for moms. Mine bundled her two babies up, and deposited us at the airport for a flight from hell—delayed, crowded, with squirmy baby and crippled back.

Determined not to repeat my last back-attack experience, a year later I began researching this book. I owe a great deal to the specialists who have taken an enormous amount of their time to educate me about why so many backs hurt. I've met hundreds of people with back pain, most more severe than mine. Yet the common bone that runs through the back stories is a lack of understanding about what makes our backs hurt. Perhaps even more pronounced and disturbing is that when we *get* an inkling of how poor posture, lifting heavy objects, and stress affects our backs, we then choose to ignore it. In some cases a trip to the chiropractor or specialist eases the pain. In others, bouncing from doctors to pain relievers to surgery brings some relief, permanent or temporary. But all who suffer from back pain want to know one thing: Will there be a cure, a revolutionary breakthrough in the twenty-first century for our back?

PART I

UNDERSTANDING CONDITIONS AND CARE OF YOUR SPINE

Chapter 1

SPINAL PHYSIOLOGY

Let's look at the lay of the land here. The average person knows more about home plumbing than his or her own body. When a leaky faucet drips, you fix it or call in an expert. Sometimes you maintain your own plumbing, and other times you dial for help. Roto-Rooter can pretty much fix anything, and if it can't be fixed, you pitch the corroded part and replace it with a shiny new one. We can't do this with our body. Sure, doctors can transplant a heart or a liver, but ultimately the responsibility for your own well-being falls squarely on your back. Many of us take better care of the plumbing under the kitchen sink than we do our own backs. A good strong backbone may conjure up images of courage and strength, but ultimately, this slinkylike structure, which conjures up images of courage and strength, governs the well-being of your entire body.

The backbone is often used to describe the most important part of an entity, and for good reason: It's this S-curved structure around which our ability to walk, run, and sleep is hinged. Our arms, legs, chest, and head all attach to the spine. And the spine affects and is affected by every movement we make. No back problem can be isolated from how the rest of our body functions. Because of this interdependence, only by understanding the whole body and how movements affect the spine can we approach back problems. This chapter will describe the basic spinal structure and how the intricate web of bone, tissue, and muscle maintains the basis for your ability to move through life.

In animals, body weight is distributed evenly on all four legs; dinosaurs or dog, the spine lies in a horizontal position. Animals may be afflicted with their own sets of problems, but back pain usually isn't among them. In human beings, however, the spine is held in a vertical position. Walking upright may have freed our ancestors to engage in myriad civilized activities, from sipping tea to carrying a bag of groceries, but it literally created a pain in our backs. Walking on two legs places an enormous strain on our spines.

The back is not made up of a single bone but is an engineering masterpiece, composed of donut-shaped bones called vertebrae. These irregular, spool-shaped structures are stacked one on top of the other. Each vertebra is separated by a ring of shock-absorbing cartilage. These disks make spinal movement possible.

Your spine is divided into five sections: the cervical, the thoracic, the lumbar, the sacrum, and the coccyx. The skeleton contains thirty-three vertebrae that extend from the base of the skull to the tailbone.

The neck contains the seven cervical vertebrae that descend from the skull to the shoulders, becoming larger as they move downward. *Cervical* is the Latin word for neck. Next comes the thoracic or upper and middle part of the spine, and it contains twelve thoracic vertebrae, moving down from the shoulder to the end of the rib cage. The lower back contains the five lumbar vertebrae, which continue from the ribs to the hips. *Lumbar* pertains to the loins, and these five lumbar vertebrae are the most substantial in the spinal cavity. Five additional vertebrae fuse together to make up the sacrum, which is held between the iliac bones of the pelvis on either side, forming the sacroiliac joints. Back problems frequently occur where the lumbar spine connects to the sacrum. Below the sacrum sits the coccyx or tailbone, consisting of four and sometimes five small vertebrae. According to one source, "coccyx" means cuckoo, because this part of the spine resembles a bird's bill.

The cervical and the lumbar vertebrae are capable of an enormous range of movement. The neck, the most flexible part of the spine, balances and supports the head, which weighs twelve to fifteen pounds. The neck never gets a rest. The thoracic spine, guarded by the rib cage and the sacrum, is not as mobile as the other parts of the back.

Keep in mind that your spinal column supports the head and allows the entire torso to bend and twist. The spinal column also protects the spinal cord, which houses a bundle of nerves, or ganglia, that connect our brain to our body. The interdependent relationship between the spinal column and the spinal cord is a wondrous, complex marvel that few of us ever think about.

Spinal Curves

Each section of the spine has a natural curve. Viewed from the side, the cervical and lumbar spines have a lordotic, or slight concave curve, and the thoracic spine has a kyphotic, or gentle convex curve (Fig. 1).

Natural curves are important. Without these curves the spine would not have the strength and resilience to act as a shock absorber during movement. The back's curves are designed to absorb shock and to facilitate the full range of motion throughout the spinal column. The natural curves act as a coiled spring to absorb force or jarring during activity. Jogging or jumping rope would be impossible without these curves. The yielding curves are the pillars of strength, resilience, and flexibility in the spine. Nonetheless, our back's flexibility is not without its own set of problems.

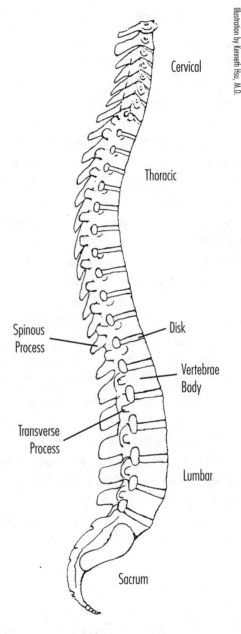

Illustration by Kenneth Hsu, M.D.

Cervical

Thoracic

Spinous Process

Disk

Vertebrae Body

Transverse Process

Lumbar

Sacrum

FIGURE 1: THE SPINAL COLUMN.

WHAT ARE VERTEBRAE?

Remember Anatomy 101, the white bony structure dangling in the lab, and the professor's lecture on the spinal column? While you snored through it, the professor probed the odd-shaped bones with a pointer, explaining that the spine was an interlocking structure of peculiar-looking bones called vertebrae. Very interesting, right? But what are vertebrae? Vertebrae are the building blocks of your spine (Fig. 2) . The twenty-four separate vertebrae are spool shaped and about an inch in height. They protect ten billion nerve cells in the spinal cord. Stacked between each vertebra is a shock absorbing disk. If we put too much pressure on a disk, it can rupture, or herniate, and may be extremely painful (we'll talk more about this in chapter 2). This vertebrae-disk combination originally supported animals that walked on all fours. Evolution changed all that.

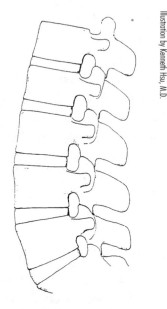

Illustration by Kenneth Hsu, M.D.

FIGURE 2: THE SPINAL VERTEBRAE.

Once man stood upright, the back vertebrae shifted and were no longer at the center of the body but toward the rear. The vertebrae are continually pulled forward—and out of alignment—by unequal weight distribution. Standing erect puts nearly a hundred pounds of pressure on the lumbar spine.

The weight-bearing lumbar vertebrae are massive. The cervical vertebrae, which support the head, are smaller. Stacked to the rear of each vertebral unit are bony projections. They extend from the rear of each vertebra to form neural arches that make up the spinal canal, which protects the delicate spinal cord. The muscles that bend and allow the spine to rotate affix to these bony projections and are called spinous and transverse processes.

FACET JOINTS

The gliding joints between the vertebrae are called facet joints or facet articulations. The little facet joints direct and limit the angle at which your spine moves. If you run your fingers down toward the low back, you can feel the bony protuberance, or spinous processes, through the skin. The bony protuberances of the joints are covered with smooth cartilage. Part of the lining nourishes and lubricates the joint. Irritation and inflammation in this area result in back pain. Irritation of the facet joints is common. The facet joints are not designed to carry excessive body weight.

INTERVERTEBRAL DISKS

Disks are thick pads of cartilage that separate adjacent vertebrae. Disks serve as shock absorbers, and you'd better take good care of them. Unlike the shock absorbers in a car, these cannot be discarded and replaced. If you have ever had a dysfunctional disk, you certainly understand what I'm talking about.

Each disk is made up of two parts: a gelatinous center called the nucleus, and an outer gristly, interwoven fibrocartilage called the annulus fibrosis. The inside of the disk is like a jelly donut, while the outer disk resembles the rings of a tree.

When young, the center or nucleus retains water. It is through the jelly-filled nucleus and bony plates of the vertebrae that the disk acquires nourishment. Constituting about a third of the length of your spine, the intervertebral disks constitute the largest organ in the body without its own blood supply. Like a sea predator, it's completely dependent on a spongylike motion to attract nutrients from adjacent tissue. The disks receive their blood supply through movement as they soak up nutrients.

When at rest, the disk expands, soaking up fluid. This increases the length of the spine as much as one inch overnight. But wake up and begin weight-bearing activity such as walking, and the fluid compresses back into the adjacent soft tissue and vertebrae. When inhibited through repetitive movement, injury, or poor posture, this mechanism and the disks become thinner and prone to injury. This can ultimately lead to degenerative disk disease.

LIGAMENTS

Ligaments are strong fibrous bands that bind the skeleton together. The ligaments of the spine hold the vertebral bones together, stabilize the spine, and protect the disks. The two major ligaments are the anterior longitudinal ligament and the posterior longitudinal ligament. These continuous bands run from the top to the bottom of the spine along the vertebral bodies, providing a structure to prevent excessive movement of the vertebral bones. This is essential, considering that the major nerves of the body run through the spine. The ligamental structure is powerful, but in a weakened or continually stressed state, it cannot support the spine.

MUSCLES

Back muscles are complex. They provide strength for movement and lengthen or constrict in response to stress. When muscles become tight or weak, as they often do at the first sign of stress or an injury, back pain may occur. A large percentage of back pain is caused by muscle strain or soft-tissue injury.

The two main muscle groups that affect the back are extensors and flexors. The extensor muscles enable us to stand up and lift objects. This group of small back muscles work cooperatively together. The extensors are attached to the rear of the spine.

The flexor muscles are in the front and include the abdominal muscles. These muscles enable us to flex, or bend forward, and are important in lifting and controlling the arch in the lower back. They encompass the gluteal muscles, beginning at the pelvis, and attach to the femur. The flexors are individual muscles that provide support for the spine. As guy wires stabilize an antenna, back muscles stabilize your spine. Imagine what happens to your back when you are not in good physical condition. Something as common as poor muscle tone or a beer belly can pull your entire body out of alignment. Misalignment puts incredible strain on the spine. Unfortunately, without any help, back muscles begin to weaken in the third decade of life, and inactivity only accelerates this process.

Running parallel to the spine are two bands called paraspinal muscles. They support the spine in an upright position, allow the spine to rotate, and influence posture. Muscle harmony is important for the spine to function properly. As with any of the flexor or extensor muscles, if you tax the paraspinals, they, too, will spasm.

NERVES

The most sensitive parts of the back are the spinal cord and its branches, called nerves. If you were to take a dime and drop it from twelve inches onto the exposed spinal cord, the result would be severe, permanent damage the equivalent of paralysis. Fortunately, the cord is encased within a strong, bony spine to protect it. The cord itself runs from the base of the brain through the spinal canal and down to the first lumbar vertebrae. The nerves exiting from the spine, called peripheral nerves, are not as sensitive to injury or compression as those within the spinal canal. The nerves that emerge from between the lumbar and sacral vertebrae run down the length of the spinal canal as they make their way to the lower lumbar and sacral regions. The strands of nerves, similar to strands of horsehair, are called *cauda equina,* or "horse's tail" in Latin. Many of these nerves are sensitive to pain. Small nerve branches also provide sensation to the ligaments, disks, and joints of the spine.

Now that you are completely schooled in what comprises a solid backbone, as well as the interdependent relationship among the vertebrae, ligaments, and muscles, uncovering the mystery in chapter 2 of why so many backs hurt may not prove to be so arcane after all.

Chapter 2

WHY SO MANY BACKS HURT

Patty dug in her car trunk to retrieve a spare tire and froze. A sharp pain took her breath away. Straightening up was out of the question. Hunched over like a cripple, Patty summoned a friend to get her home and into bed. In a few days the pain dissipated to a dull ache. Bad move, sore back. Feeling better, Patty concluded to be prudent when changing tires. Patty resumed her daily activities. A few months later while pumping gas her back went out again. Bad car karma, or something seriously wrong with her back?

A trip to a chiropractor confirmed a pulled muscle. Wanting more information, she saw a general practitioner, who prescribed a round of painkillers and rest. While zoning out on drugs, another painful back episode derailed her life. She pitched the pills, which caused drowsiness, and decided to tough it out. Pragmatically, Patty reasoned, this back stuff couldn't go on forever. She was wrong. The bouts of pain continued with such severity that Patty missed weeks of work. She felt doomed; what else could go wrong with her life? Two months later, while stopped at a red light, the car behind her plunged into the backseat and her head shot forward and then back again. Relief was a long time coming. Patty saw an orthopedist, who diagnosed whiplash and suggested a CAT scan. A CAT scan for whiplash, quipped Patty. Her orthopedist suspected other problems. The scan showed moderately severe disk disease, with arthritis in the neck and lower back. His recommendation: surgery, and don't wait too long.

Nope, no surgery, resolved Patty, who'd heard enough horror stories about failed back surgery to fill a locker room. Weeks melted into months. Patty relied on physical therapy to get her through the long, painful days. Relief was temporary, but it was something. Confused and disgusted, Patty became a chronic-back-pain statistic.

Patty's back saga started at age twenty-three. Eleven years later, she still is not pain free. but her sojourn through the maze of practitioners ended in good fortune. She discovered a chiropractor who was able to both educate her and help her control her back pain. He encouraged her to learn about her back problems, designed an exercise program for her, and in times of distress counseled her. Patty considers herself a lucky statistic.

THE PAINFUL CERTAINTY

The back has one pronounced certainty: Many different conditions make it hurt. Back pain is epidemic, puzzling, and frustrating.

The majority of back pain is insidious and not linked to any one traumatic event. As in Patty's case, it strikes suddenly, often in the midst of a routine activity most of the time. She still has degenerative disk disease which flares up. The pain can be low-grade or chronic, limiting activity. The average back demands one thing when it's aching: a quick cure.

Back sufferers tend to diagnose their own back problems. In many instances they are right, but just as many times, self-diagnosis is incorrect. True, 80 percent of the time, someone with backache will be pain free within six weeks, and within three months after the first onset of pain, 90 percent will have recovered completely. Most lower back pain cures itself. Unfortunately, however, the likelihood that a person will suffer another back episode is very high.

Back problems may strike precipitously, but most backaches involve lifestyle issues. Usually it is we who are the culprits when our backs revolt. We, after all, take advantage of our backs. Poor postural habits, obesity, and flabby lifestyle all reflect on the landscape of our back. Loping through life with our head down, shoulders rounded, and stomachs protruding predisposes disks, joints, and muscles to injury and also speeds up the degenerative process of the spine.

Michelle is a classic example. A forty-five-year-old veterinarian, Michelle moved though life without much physical discomfort. She had had her share of psychological pain, however, starting with the death of her mother when she was four. Her loss caused her to sink into a shell like a tortoise. A bright child, Michelle excelled in school but was painfully shy. Although she received honor after honor, she never held her head high. For nearly forty years, Michelle walked with her head down and shoulders rounded. It wasn't until she hunched over a cat in her clinic that a mild back spasm caused her to stand up. She took a few aspirins, but as the weeks went by the pain worsened. Her doctor took one look at her posture and explained the relationship between spinal misalignment and good posture. Michelle could visually see her problem in the mirror. Unfortunately, despite the library of books on the subject, bad habits die hard.

Arthur H. White, orthopedic surgeon and a pioneer in the back field, promotes the concept of early back-education in schools, a kind of cradle-to-diploma approach. Imagine learning how to sit, stand, and lift—all before your first date! It just might make back pain as passé as the horse and buggy. In fact, White is convinced that whoever has the foresight to add back education to the curriculum will own the back field.

Back pain is the leading cause of absenteeism and lost productivity in America. By some estimates, back pain goes well over the $50-million-a-year mark when medical care, worker's compensation payments, and time lost from the job are combined. Some estimates move closer to a whopping $90 million.

But again, back problems are mainly lifestyle issues. Let's examine the most common back ailments and their cause. Stress tops the list.

Stress . . . As American as Apple Pie

Americans may not know why their backs give them problems, but they can certainly tell you what causes stress in their lives: deadlines, job changes, divorce, new babies, disgruntled bosses. Stress is as American as apple pie.

Everyone endures personal stress in life. It's like oxygen; we can't seem to live without it. Some of us manage our stress rather well, while others explode when things don't go so smoothly. We blame our stress on unexpected situations, like an unwelcome guest at dinnertime. But once we examine our hectic schedules, the obvious appears: Our stress is self-inflicted. We choose what's important in our lives and decide how much to cram into twenty-four hours. Leisure time becomes a marathon event, leaving little chance for relaxation.

Sometimes we cannot foresee a particularly stressful situation, such as a death in the family, or a sudden job layoff. But as the two following examples indicate, people can handle stress in very different ways.

Joanne, a forty-year-old mother of two children, lost her husband to cancer last year. It was a shock to everyone. Healthy and in the prime of life, her husband was the ideal candidate to beat cancer. He didn't, and his premature loss left both his family and their finances shattered. Joanne confided that after her husband's death, other stressful situations seemed trivial. She found solace in her children, friends, and tai chi.

"I have been a tai chi instructor for nearly eighteen years. Practicing tai chi helped me balance my emotions and kept my body strong. I even went to tai chi camp prior to my husband's death. I knew it would center me enough to face the inevitable. I also needed to get away from the house for a few days. I let friends come in and cook, take care of the house, and help me get my finances in order. I cried a lot, joined a grief group, and I won't tell you life isn't stressful—every minute with two children is a challenge. But this is life, as messy as it is, and I can either accept it, and attempt to flow with it, or let it break my back."

Linda's stress is of a much different sort. Linda waited six years to remodel the kitchen in her Victorian flat. Construction began vigorously and slowed to a snail's pace. The contents of her kitchen lined her hallway. Her life revolved around the whims of contractors, inspectors, and builders who didn't show up. She lived without a kitchen for months. Her neck and back clumped into spasm after spasm, and she got sick. Linda will tell you that she's intense, likes to get things done now, and doesn't handle stress well. With the hearth of her living situation in shambles, Linda's back and neck would not fare well until the kitchen got back together. And Linda had no outlet for her stress.

Whether it's a death, home construction, or a toothache, any unforeseen situation can translate into a bout of back pain. Stress cuts off oxygen to the blood supply. Muscles ball up and go into spasm. Life can literally become a pain in the back.

In his book *Freedom from Back Pain*, Edward A. Abraham talks about the anatomy of stress. He concludes that stress is not always a negative force, but that it's our perception that determines whether a situation is negative or positive. In either case, our body responds to a stressful situation by energizing itself beyond our average expectation. Meeting a deadline is stressful, working all night on a project we love is stressful—both are accomplishments our body gears up for by releasing adrenaline and other stress hormones into our bloodstream. We gear up for the challenge and complete it. If the body can rest completely upon completion of the deadline or project, it has a chance to refresh and recover for the next challenge. But unfortunately, many of us do not program a sufficient amount of relaxation into our lives, and so we lug our body from one stressful situation to another. If stress cannot be eliminated through physical activity or relaxation, it builds like a chemical toxin in the body. And it results in negativity, mental confusion, and depression.

I Was Born Under the Sign of Stress

In the 1960s, cardiologist Myer Friedman came up with the now-familiar term Type A behavior. He found that Type A behavior literally predisposed people to heart attacks. Guess what? A lot of Type As also have bad backs.

How do you know if you're a classic Type A personality? Do you zigzag in and out of traffic on the freeway, impatient to arrive thirty seconds before the car in front of you? Are you always in a rush? Do you interrupt conversations and harbor a lot of anxiety? Do you have a short fuse, become impatient, and hate standing in lines? Yes? You were born under the sign of Type A. Watch your heart and your back.

You may not be able to modify your personality, but your behavior is another story. If stress seems to be the story of your day, here are some prescriptives for taking a load off your back.

Stress Thermometer: Hot or Cold?

Find out where your trouble spots are on the stress thermometer. Do you have difficulty prioritizing or deciding what to do first? Do you feel overwhelmed at work, with family, or life in general? Do you do it all, or are you willing to delegate tasks? Are you competitive, or do you work cohesively with others? Be honest.

After examining your character, assemble your priorities. Make two lists: one of things that are important in your life, and the other of things you spend time doing. Compare them. If what's important is getting overwhelmed by what you spend time doing, make some adjustments so that you can get on with what gives you pleasure.

The late Norman Cousins in his book *Anatomy of an Illness* talks about how vital laughter, a sense of humor, and doing what makes you happy is to a healthy body and soul. Your back is a big part of your anatomy, so be kind to it, lighten its load, and watch your stress thermometer drop.

Back Up and Cultivate a Little Joy in Your Life

You don't need a high-tech course in stress reduction to alleviate back pain. But you will have to alter your lifestyle. If work is a pain in the back, cut back if possible. Leave your work at the office. The back wasn't designed for a sixty-hour-a-week sit-down job. Take a walk. And if you absolutely cannot avoid job stress, make sure your leisure activity is *leisurely*.

Engage in a hobby, something you love that brings you joy. Joy balances your stress level. Whether hunkering down among the radishes and lettuce in your garden, dancing the cha-cha, or curling up with tea and a good murder mystery, doing what you love balances stress and it makes your back happy too.

Attitude

Adjust your attitude. Stress is as much internal as external. If you cannot say no and feel your life is stacking up like an overloaded in-basket, get some assertiveness training. Take control. Statistics show that individuals who go through life feeling victimized by work relationships and family have a slow recovery when it comes to back problems.

Laying of the Hands

For centuries, people in Asia and Europe have used massage to relax. In the last two decades, massage has taken on a life of its own in this country. Though we'll cover massage more thoroughly in an upcoming chapter, let me just say now that massage is invaluable for relieving tension, alleviating fatigue, and instilling relaxation. If your neck or back problems stem from stressful situations you struggle to get a handle on, try massage.

Peace of Mind

How about a little peace of mind for your back? Meditation may not guarantee nirvana, but it's a great tension buster. Why meditate for back problems? Because ultimately what is good for the head is good for the body. You cannot relax your body without first unwinding the clock upstairs.

Meditation involves stealing a few quiet moments to focus your attention inwardly. You don't need a guru, although some find taking a group class helpful. Meditation can be difficult for the mind that is always turned on, cluttered with chatter. The goal of meditation is to quiet the mind, and this can be a shock to many first-time meditators.

The easiest way to meditate is to find a quiet spot and take the phone off the hook and shut off your beepers. Loosen your tie, kick off your shoes, put on unbinding clothes, and sit comfortably in a chair or cross-legged on the floor. Sit straight, but not as if you've got a pipe running through your body. If you're in a quagmire with your back, support it with a pillow and don't stay in any position that is uncomfortable. When I'm stressed to the max, my lower back revolts. Lord knows, writing a book takes a toll on the head and body. After too much time at the computer, the last thing I want to do is sit and meditate. But I recognize the benefits of relaxing, so I lie on the floor on my back, legs and arms spread slightly apart. I tense the entire body, moving up from my feet to my face. I flex the legs, I scrunch up my face like a prune, then I release and relax. After I've tensed and released my torso, I close my eyes and do the old get-yourself-to-sleep trick. I command my feet, legs, pelvic area, arms, hands, shoulders, stomach, back, chest, and face and head to relax. And they do. All through the relaxation, I breathe slowly. Don't worry, thoughts love to clutter the landscape of the mind—*What's for dinner? I forgot to pick up the baby! Must water the plants.* Bat those thoughts off court, and just continue to breathe and breathe. This fifteen-minute little gem is one of the best relaxation techniques I know.

If self relaxation proves too difficult, there are hundreds of tapes that foster relaxation. Even classical music will do it.

Lube Your Spirits

To maintain a healthy back, lube your spirits. Watch a sunset, hug your child, take a two-day retreat to a mountain cabin, walk in the woods, take a vacation. A vacation is a surefire antidote to stress. Remember, the back is not an entity all its own. Whatever aids your mind, body, and spirit to rid itself of stress ultimately pleases the back.

So now that you're a master of stress reduction, and your back is humming along like a fine-tuned Mercedes, what else could cause your back to downshift into spasms? Something as minor as lifting your golden retriever or your year-old infant. Lifting is the second leading cause of back pain.

Lifting

Lifting puts stress on your spinal structure. It puts tremendous pressure on your vertebrae. We lift windows, groceries, children, and golf bags—you name it, we lift it. And we never stop to think about how we lift an object; we just give it the old heave-ho. Did you ever watch passengers at an airport scramble between terminals or run to catch planes with luggage slung over their shoulders for a month-long safari? This is a real lesson in how not to treat your back.

If you work in a profession that requires you to lift, you understand that lifting puts enormous strain on the back. If your job involves nursing, construction, heavy equipment, child care, or handling baggage, mastering the technique of lifting is paramount to a healthy back.

There is a secret to lifting: Hold the object close to you. The farther away from you the object is, the more pressure on your vertebrae. Distribute weight evenly, and always bend your knees so that you reduce your distance from the ground. Squat or bend on one knee, then slowly rise. Always use your legs to lift, not your back. Never twist when lifting. If you must turn, use your feet. *Never lean over or bend from the waist to pick up anything.* Never carry a child on your hip. Parents often make the mistake of reaching for a child like a sack of groceries. According to Dr. Mary Schatz, author of *Basic Back Care, a Doctor's Gentle Yoga Program for Back and Neck Relief,* holding a 20-pound child or grocery bag transmits a 300-pound load to the spine. Imagine what lifting a 40-pound suitcase or piece of furniture does to your back.

Is Your Job an Occupational Hazard?

In 1975 Hank injured his back lifting and loading heavy freight. He managed with the pain. A few months after the incident, Hank was dressing for work when a severe back pain stopped him in his tracks. He couldn't move. Never having had a medical problem in his young life, Hank didn't know what to do. His roommate took him to the emergency room. Writhing in pain, he was given papers to fill out. The receptionist asked his religious preference. Hank glared across the desk and declared he needed medical attention, not bureaucracy. He sat for what seemed like hours before he was seen by a doctor. He was given drugs. The doctor suspected a herniated disk and made an appointment for Hank to see an orthopedist. Hank went to bed until his appointment a few days later.

"The orthopedic doctor was a stroke of good luck," says Hank. "The X ray showed two herniated disks, but the doctor cautioned against surgery and recommended a more conservative approach. He felt surgery should be the last resort. He gave me exercises and sent me to a physical therapist. He cautioned that we may not be able to reverse the problem, but we could keep it under control if I actively participated through exercise and rest when needed."

Hank went for two years without another incident. He became a pilot and was based in Miami when a second back episode, similar to the first, put him in the hospital for six weeks.

"This was a nightmare. The doctor ordered pelvic traction, chatted about airplanes, but didn't have the time to actually discuss my back. I felt that the entire staff saw dollar signs. The medical experience in Miami was the antithesis of my medical experience in California. After six weeks on my back, I left the hospital."

Several months later Hank returned to California, where his back pain teetered between manageable and intense. Sometimes he slept sitting up. In 1981 he had another painful back episode. By this time he had done enough research to know something had to be done. He returned to his orthopedic specialist. Both Hank and his doctor wanted to pursue the least invasive route. Hank flew to Vancouver, Canada, to try the experimental chymopapain injection, which in 1981 was not yet available in the United States. Hank had a CAT scan, which confirmed the two herniated disks.

Hank's chymopapain treatment was a dramatic success. His pain scale plunged. Prior to his treatment, on a scale of 100 to 0, 30 was his best day and 2 his worst day. After chymopapain, he rated 99 as his best day and 85 his worst day.

"I realize chymopapain didn't and doesn't work for everyone. In my case, it was part of the answer. Today, almost twenty years after my first back attack, I exercise daily. Exercise is not an option but a necessity to keep my back in shape. I have a great orthopedist who nurtured me down the right path. I'm lucky."

Today, Hank is still in the profession he loves. He water skis, snow skis, hikes, and sits in the cockpit with relatively little back pain. He doesn't consider his job an occupational hazard; he understands how to take care of his back.

Occupations can be unkind and stressful to the back. Certain jobs, however, are more hazardous than others: If you stand in one place, drive, lift, or sit, you're a candidate for back pain. Now you see why so many Americans suffer from back problems at some point in their lifetimes. Occupational change isn't an option for most; learning how to create a better work environment and taking care of your back in the workplace is.

If you must stand, by all means stand straight. As I mentioned earlier, poor posture is the kiss of death to a healthy back. Standing in one place for hours is also uncomfortable for your back. If you're in a job that demands staying on your two feet all day, get a small stool approximately six inches in height and place one leg on the stool while keeping the other leg straight. Alternate legs. If a stool is out of the question, stand with knees slightly bent. Try to be aware of your center of gravity when standing.

Anyone who drives long distances understands that car seats are not designed with the human spine in mind. Even a weekend trip can be unkind to your back. If you have the time, money, and inclination, research your car before purchasing it. Test-drive it for comfort as well as endurance.

Before you take to the road, position your seat so that you can easily reach the wheel. Accordingly, don't strain to reach the brake, clutch, or accelerator. Adjust the seat for height, maintaining your knees slightly higher than your hips. Stop frequently and walk or stretch. I can't emphasize this enough. If your car seat provides inadequate support for the lower back, try a rolled-up towel, lumbar support, or car-seat insert. Don't slouch behind the wheel. Avoid twisting or reaching behind. Driving a car for a healthy back is as much about don't as do.

Are you plugged into the electronic superhighway? Do you sit at a computer terminal? If the answer is yes, chances are you've already logged on to sedentary work habits. The average American sits most of the day and often into the evening. This, coupled with inferior chairs and poor posture, adds up to one of the leading causes of industrial back pain. Sitting for an extended period of time stresses the back. Sitting is especially painful if you have disk disease.

I hate to sound like your mother, but sit straight! Don't round your shoulders forward. Sit with your knees higher than your hips; make sure the lumbar spine is supported. Try sitting with your buttocks all the way back in the chair, not on the edge of your chair.

Some chairs offer levers to tilt the seat forward. Redesign your work environment so that you have an adjustable seat that allows your feet to be flat on the floor, allows the thighs to rest comfortably, and leaves the knees bent at about a 90-degree angle. Don't forget to support the lumbar spine with an adjustable backrest. Choose a seat that is wide enough to move around in and that has armrests. Get up and stretch; do not remain seated for long periods of time. Pull off the road from that superhighway every hour and stretch or walk around.

Having a modicum of control over your environment empowers you and allows you to take charge of your back pain. But often you have no control over events that catapult your back and neck into spasms and a very long journey rife with pain. Whiplash is one of those unexpected journeys. It makes you wish you'd never left the house.

WHIPLASH

Over 60 percent of the population consults a physician for a lifetime of headache or neck pain. Injury due to neck sprains and strain can affect the arm, shoulder, jaw, or upper back. Individuals often seek medical treatment for cervical injury resulting from whiplash. If you've never experienced whiplash, chances are pretty good you know someone who has. Twenty to 60 percent of car accidents result in this condition.

Whiplash is a popular term for cervical strain with separation of one or more vertebrae. Whiplash occurs when the head and neck are violently jerked, usually when a vehicle has been rear-ended or is in a head-on collision.

To understand what happens with whiplash, let's look at the function of your neck. The neck does more than simply connect the head to the rest of your body. The neck's anatomy houses many fragile parts. The vertebrae and joints make up the spinal column, and the muscles and ligaments help support and move your head and neck. In a whiplash, the forceful impact most commonly affects the ligaments, muscles, and nerves at the base of the skull. Because the spinal cord is also encased in the neck, whiplash can create a myriad of problems.

Whiplash turns your head into a powerful force, hurling the neck past its normal range of motion. Whiplash unbalances the anatomy of your neck. When the neck experiences such a trauma, loss of balance, numbness in the extremities, and nausea, although not necessarily symptomatic of whiplash, may result. To add insult to injury, whiplash victims are often not taken seriously. Monetary vengeance, greedy lawyers, and insurance companies have given whiplash victims a bad rap.

Whiplash may occur instantly or come on a few days after an accident. Treatment may be arduous, but it should begin immediately. Here you have an array of specialists to choose from: chiropractors, physiotherapists, orthopedic specialists, osteopaths, and acupuncturists. You may not be happy with some of the therapies, such as strapping your head into a halter or traction. The most effective treatment usually combines hot and cold packs and manipulation. Manipulation stretches the tissue and unlocks joints. If manipulation is your doctor's choice, the body should be warmed first by massage. And massage itself may help. All these may be used with intermittent traction. Severe whiplash is rehabilitated with physical therapy, and a brace may be required.

How do you prevent whiplash? You may not always be able to prevent an accident, but you can make sure you're doing your best to buckle up safely. Always wear a seatbelt. A well-padded headrest at the right height might minimize impact upon collision. And all those rear brake lights mounted in the center rear window of the car in front of you are there to alert you to slow down and possibly stop.

UNNATURAL ACCIDENTS

Accidents account for the majority of spinal paralysis, and they happen without warning. When actor Christopher Reeve fell in a freak horseback riding accident in 1995, he severed the nerves in his spinal column. Reeve was a conscientious rider who never took risks on his horse. Yet, the horse Reeve was riding refused to jump, halted, and hurled the 215-pound rider head-first to the ground, shattering his top two cervical vertebrae, and paralyzing Reeve from the neck down. In 1996, twenty-three-year-old Detroit Lions football player Reggie Brown dislocated his two top vertebrae when his helmet awkwardly struck another player. The accident cut off the neurological pathway that controlled Brown's breathing.

What happened to Reggie Brown and Christopher Reeve is what athletes fear most—an injury that will end their career and one that could mean paralysis. Neither Reeve's nor Brown's accident are everyday back traumas; yet when such an accident does occur, it results in serious psychological and physical trauma—a near brush with death and the loss of a physical mobility we all take for granted.

HERNIATED DISK

The infamous herniated intervertebral disk is the most common cause of low back pain associated with a defined structural abnormality. Contrary to popular belief, herniated disks don't appear overnight, although the onset of pain can be sudden.

Audrey, for example, never had a back problem in her life. One day while leaning over her seat at a Giants game a twinge of pain pricked her ankle. She ignored it. A few days later in the first inning of another game, a sharp pain seared through her low back, down the left buttock, and into the hip. One minute Audrey was standing at Candlestick Park cheering for the Giants, and the next moment she was slumped over her seat, unable to move. Thinking she had pulled a muscle, her husband drove her to her chiropractor. X rays and an MRI were ordered. In 1990 Audrey had a hysterectomy for carcinoma. The chiropractor wanted to rule out cancer. Audrey visited the chiropractor daily. Nothing worked. Massage gave only temporary relief. If she wasn't at the doctors, Audrey spent her days and nights flat on her back. Her chiropractor sent her to an orthopedic surgeon, who gave her an epidural injection to shrink the swelling. The pain dissipated, but the epidural left her foot and ankle numb. The orthopedist considered surgery. Audrey declined and began searching for another doctor. A friend suggested she try an osteopath.

"The first time I visited him, I didn't feel any difference, and I began to feel like a failed experiment. I continued treatment, and to my surprise, after the fourth visit the numbness disappeared. The doctor said I had probably had a bulging disk for years prior to pain. He restructured my entire body with gentle motions of pressure and pulling. He'd pull my leg out and move it. He understood that the pain radiating down my buttocks sent shock waves through my entire body. Because I had spent so much time on my back, my neck was a mess. We talked about posture and stress. He gave me exercises. I did them religiously. In two months, I was pain free. To date, I've never had a reoccurrence and hope I never do."

What happened to Audrey's disk is not uncommon. Remember that the disk is made up of two parts, a center and an outer layer. When it bulges between two vertebrae, the soft jelly center, the nucleus pulposus, protrudes or spurts out. It's the shock absorber between the vertebral bodies.

As we age, the nucleus loses fluid, volume, and resiliency. The entire disk structure becomes susceptible to irritation and trauma. If there are repeated small injuries to the disk, tears develop in the body of the annulus, the thick, rubberlike padding that surrounds the nucleus pulposus. These small injuries can occur from twisting, sitting incorrectly, or lifting. When a disk degenerates due to age or injury, weak points develop on the normally tough outer layer. Pressure on the disk causes the jellylike center to seep out, causing the disk to lose even more of its elasticity. When the protrusion presses on a nerve root, pinching it against the bone, pain results elsewhere in the body. This is what happened to Audrey.

The term *slipped disk* is often used to describe this painful problem. Disks, however, are anchored in place and do not slip. The disk does not move back into place; instead, scar tissue forms around it. If stressed continually, the tissue weakens further and the slightest activity—a sneeze or cough—may cause the disk to rupture. It's painful, and if a nerve root is irritated in any one place, the entire root is affected. Sometimes stiffness accompanies this pain. Tingling and numbness in the buttocks and leg is a pretty good indication that you've herniated a disk.

The course of treatment for a herniated disk depends on who you see. Surgery is not usually indicated; progressive practitioners tend to favor a conservative approach. This can include taking painkillers, such as anti-inflammatories, a few days in bed, physical therapy, applying ice, and readjustment of such lifestyle habits as sitting, walking, and lifting. Depending on the damaged disk, epidural injections to relieve swelling and dissolve the disk may be an option. Surgery is rare. A word of caution about surgery for a herniated disk: Always seek a second opinion, and exhaust all other possibilities before embarking on such a course. Chapter 10 will discuss further the surgery dilemma that faces many individuals with herniated disks.

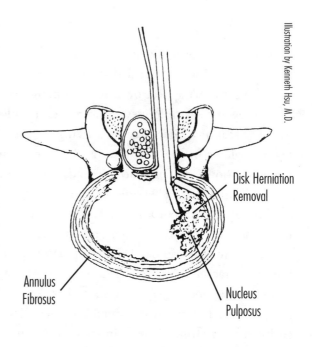

Illustration by Kenneth Hsu, M.D.

Disk Herniation Removal

Annulus Fibrosus

Nucleus Pulposus

FIGURE 3: DISK HERNIATION REMOVAL.

SCIATICA

When a ruptured disk presses on a nerve root in the lower back, causing sharp pains to radiate in the buttocks and through the leg to the foot, it causes sciatica. Sciatica might appear like a pins-and-needle sensation in your leg. You may feel a slight numbness or tingling near the buttocks, which abates after walking. A serious bout of sciatica may erupt into a throbbing, shooting pain in the back and legs; movement may be excruciating.

Sciatica involves the sciatic nerve. This nerve group, the longest in your body, runs from the lower back through the buttock and thigh, down to the knee, and on to the foot. The roots of each nerve originate among the bones of the lumbar and sacral vertebrae and connect the spinal cord with the outside of the thigh, hamstrings, and muscles in the lower leg and feet. Sciatica can lead to muscle weakness.

Two of every five people will suffer a bout of sciatica at some time in their life. Most have low back pain with sciatica, and for women the discomfort may be worse during their menstrual period. According to *The New England Journal of Medicine*, there is a high correlation between sciatica and job dissatisfaction and depression. But you don't need to be unhappy at work to suffer from an episode of sciatica. Sciatica may be brought on by fractures, tumors, infections, and pregnancy, but the primary cause involves a herniated disk pressing on one of the nerve roots.

Sciatica due to a herniated nucleus pulposus is problematic and painful. Although the majority of people suffering with sciatica recover with conservative treatment, 10 to 15 percent need surgery. Epidural corticosteroid injections are often used to treat sciatica, but while these may afford short-term improvement in pain and sensory deficits, a study reported in June 1997 of *The New England Journal of Medicine* noted that this treatment offered no significant benefit nor does it reduce the need for surgery.

Sciatica comes on suddenly. Pain is often felt on one side only and may be aggravated by sneezing or coughing. Lower back pain is usually present.

Who you see and how severe your sciatica is will dictate treatment. An acupuncturist will concentrate on points of pain with needles. A chiropractor will free the tight muscles, a general practitioner might prescribe an anti-inflammatory, and an osteopath will use gentle soft-tissue massage and positioning prior to manipulation. If sciatica is the result of a herniated disk—and often sciatica and a herniated disk go hand in hand—treatment follows the route of a herniated disk.

FACET JOINT PROBLEMS

Take your finger and reach around to the center of your back. Run your fingers down toward the lower back. Those bony projections you feel through the skin are called the spinous process. On either side of the spinous process are facet joints, which serve as hinges between each vertebra above and below. In theory, the disk should function as a perfect little unit, humming along without problems. But once you stress or injure any part of the disk, a gradual chain reaction results. Facet joints are not designed to carry excessive weight, and when this occurs, the strain causes them to move closer together. As the two parts of the facets rub together, the cartilage eventually wears rough, causing irritation, and in turn, pain and discomfort. While this is not an overnight process, a sudden twist, or even turning the wrong way in bed, can aggravate facet pain. Furthermore, if ligaments in the spine lose strength, this affects the facet joints, because they rely on other spinal ligaments for support. In general, facet point problems have degenerative changes, but it is possible to injure facet joints in an accident or trauma, like a broken neck. The disk and two facet joints make up the motion segment of the spine, allowing the spine to be flexible and strong.

What causes ligaments to sag? Poor posture, for starters. People with poor posture do not use their muscles to support their spine. Spinal ligaments take over this task, then, and over time stretch and become loose, incapable of stabilizing the vertebrae alone. When the spinal ligaments lose their tautness from overwork, the muscles must step in, flex, and compensate for the damaged ligaments. The ability of the muscles to take charge depends on their strength and coordination, which is usually poor in this situation. Ligaments cannot fully repair themselves. Severe ligament damage usually must be repaired surgically, removing torn sections and replacing them with other tissue.

PIRIFORMIS SYNDROME

The roots of sciatica aren't always linked to the back. The piriformis muscle, located deep in the buttocks, can, in rare cases, entrap the sciatic nerve, resulting in debilitating pain.

But when the piriformis muscle entraps the sciatic nerve, which runs from the lower spine down the back of the leg to the back of the lower calf, searing pain results.

The piriformis syndrome can strike anyone, and it usually occurs after a fall or blow to the buttocks. If misdiagnosed and improperly treated, pain may persist for months. Piriformis is sometimes mistaken for disk disease, or confused with gynecological or pelvic problems. The best tool for diagnosing piriformis syndrome is a physical examination by a doctor. While many doctors misdiagnose the piriformis syndrome, the muscle can be felt directly by a rectal examination. Diagnostic tests such as a CAT scan are usually a waste of time and money here.

Pain typically occurs in the upper buttock, usually on one side. Pain radiates down the thigh, sometimes to the lower leg, back, or groin. Sitting and crouching aggravate the pain. Treatment for piriformis syndrome leans toward the conservative side. Transrectal massage, heat, ultrasound, diathermy, and physical therapy commonly alleviate the problem. Injections and, rarely, surgery can help. Ask your doctor or physical therapist to teach you how to exercise, stretch, and relax the piriformis muscle so that it won't clamp onto the sciatic nerve.

SPINAL STENOSIS

Spinal stenosis is a narrowing of the spinal canal. The nerves and the spinal cord irritate and swell as the canal shrinks. There are two types of spinal stenosis: central and lateral.

Central stenosis occurs when your spinal canal is narrower than normal in a specific area. The condition is sometimes congenital. If the nerves become crammed and irritated in the canal, leg and back pain result, especially with walking and standing. Sometimes the pain is mild, in other cases severe. If you can ride a bike without difficulty but have pain in your legs when walking, you might have spinal stenosis.

Lateral stenosis is a narrowing of the intervertebral space at the sides of the vertebra. This space, called intervertebral foramen, is when the nerve root exits. Osteophytes are irregular overgrowths of bone that grow on the spine to protect shrinking disks. Osteophytes are the most common cause of lateral spinal stenosis. If encroachment is minimal, the stenosis may not be noticeable. But when a nerve root is actually being pinched, surgery may be indicated.

The *goal* of decompression surgery is to enlarge the spinal canal and relieve pressure on the nerves. Laminectomy or laminotory are the *procedures* used to achieve this. During this procedure, a portion of the bony arches of one or more vertebrae is removed to relieve compression of the nerves. If an entire segment of the vertebrae is removed, this is called a laminectomy. If only a portion is removed, this is a laminotomy procedure. The surgery does not, however, alter the ongoing degenerative arthritis.

The normal degenerative process that affects all of our bones is the most common cause of stenosis, although surgery, an injury, or a bone condition like Paget's disease can also contribute to this condition.

Spinal stenosis symptoms appear over time and are usually mild. Early warning signs include a vague, unusual feeling in the legs, a rubbery sensation, or leg pain brought on by walking or standing, due to the fact that the space for nerves has been made smaller.

Bending over or sitting will ease the pain, since these positions enlarge the spinal canal. As the condition worsens, pain may occur while sitting or sleeping.

Because stenosis is degenerative in nature, time is its enemy. Typically, pain increases and mobility decreases if spinal degeneration accelerates.

Early symptoms may be managed by exercise or a support brace that holds the spine in a flexed position, enlarging the space for the nerves and decreasing spinal motion. Symptoms may be temporarily eased with rest, ice or heat, or a TENS unit, a self-applied electrical stimulation to the nerve that blocks pain in some cases. An epidural—an injection of powerful anti-inflammatory steroids, combined with a local anesthetic—is also an option. This has been known to ease symptoms for varying periods of time.

Spinal stenosis is not difficult to diagnose with a CAT scan, MRI, or myelogram; an X ray, however, will typically not confirm the condition.

OSTEOPHYTES, OR BONE SPURS

Bone spurs are irregular overgrowths of bone on the spine that are produced to help stabilize a degenerating disk. These alterations produce major stiffness and backaches in older people. They can be painful and cause pressure on the nerves and cervical spinal cord, especially if the canal is narrow. Something as minor as walking can produce symptoms. Pressure on the cervical spinal cord may be treated surgically.

Bone spurs do not disappear or go away unless bones bridge or grow back together spontaneously, which is extremely rare.

LEG DISCREPANCY

Something as simple as unequal leg length can result in back pain. The discrepancy creates an uneven pelvis, and the spine tilts to compensate. If the leg discrepancy is not an anatomical abnormality, it can be treated by using a lift inside the shoe of the shorter leg, or with bodywork.

You usually cannot detect a leg discrepancy by looking in a mirror, but an examination by an orthopedist will usually unmask the problem.

OBESITY

Obesity, which afflicts thirty-four million Americans, increases weight on the spine and pressure on the disks. A large stomach pulls the spine forward and out of alignment, increasing the chances of back strain. The more weight the back supports, the more likely it is to revolt.

Since obesity plays a major role in spinal stress, dieting and exercise are the two best avenues for realigning such a back. Bad nutritional habits and sedentary habits may be hard to change, but with a good weight-loss and exercise program, pounds will eventually disappear.

Jack had a family legacy of obesity. His parents were heavy, and his father died of a heart attack; his mother of a stroke. Jack never exercised, and putting away a huge meal was a daily obsession. Five years ago, Jack started having back pain. He walked, did tai chi, went to the chiropractor, yet the pain became semichronic.

When Jack was forty years old, his mother died. Her death touched off his health button. He joined a gym, gave up drinking coke and pizza for lunch, and began paying attention to his diet. In six months, Jack lost his belly and sixty big pounds. He's in great shape, and his back has never been better.

SPONDYLOLYSIS AND SPONDYLOLISTHESIS

Spondylolysis is present in approximately 5 percent of the population. Because pain is not usually present until later years, those afflicted with this condition often are unaware of it.

Most spondylolysis is not congenital but acquired and is detectable in later stages via X rays. Spondylolysis can become a source of chronic low back pain and in extreme cases lead to surgery.

This condition is thought to be a stress fracture that develops in the pars interarticularis of one or several of the vertebrae, creating a painful local inflammation. Over time and ongoing stresses, the ligaments and muscles that help hold the vertebral body in place may become stretched. A vertebra may slip partially or fully off the vertebra below, and this may result in pinched nerves and severe pain.

The defect acts like a loose hinge, so that over time, ligaments and muscles may stretch and weaken, allowing the entire vertebral body to slide forward. The sliding of the vertebral body is a condition known as spondylolisthesis.

Mild cases of spondylolysis and spondylolisthesis are common and usually not painful. Recommended treatment is to strengthen back muscles and avoid lifting heavy objects. If this does not work, surgery may have to be performed to fuse the loose vertebrae.

SPINA BIFIDA

Thirty-two-year-old Julia expected a healthy delivery with her second child. Seconds after her daughter was born, her expectations turned to shock as she heard the word *spina bifida* between newborn cries and a flurry of medical activity. She remembers seeing the lump on her daughter's back, then hearing doctors talking about bladder problems and difficulty walking. Then her daughter, Celia, was whisked away to surgery, the first of many, on her tiny spine.

Spina bifida affects about 1,500 babies per year in the United States. One out of every thousand babies born in the United States has spina bifida, the second most common birth defect after Down's syndrome. An unborn baby's spine normally closes before birth, but with spina bifida, the vertebral canal does not close, for reasons not clearly understood. There is speculation that spina bifida results from a combination of heredity, environment, or a folic acid deficiency, but evidence is still circumstantial. Julia took prenatal vitamins with folic acid, but her research revealed that spina bifida appears more in countries with high pollution rates. No one, however, really knows who is at risk or why it occurs.

A blood test for spina bifida is given in the sixteenth week of pregnancy to determine the level of alpha fetoprotein (AFP)—a chemical found in the amniotic fluid, the baby's blood, and the pregnant mother's blood—to detect spina bifida. Julia had the blood test, and her AFP came back normal. Her daughter's spina bifida was not detected because a layer of skin covering the opening in her daughter's spine prevented the spinal fluid from leaking into the amniotic fluid and elevating the AFP level in Julia's blood. Because her AFP level was okay, Julia was not given an amniocentesis or ultrasound. An amniocentesis will detect spina bifida. A combination of a blood test, ultrasound, and amniocentesis can detect approximately 90 percent of neural-tube defects.

Coccygeal Pain

Coccygeal pain refers to pain emanating from the coccyx, or the base of the spine. One cause of coccygeal pain is falling and hitting the tailbone on the floor or a hard surface. Such pain can be difficult to get rid of, but it rarely creates a drastic problem. Try removing pressure from the area by sitting on a soft pillow or displacing your body weight so it is not directly on the bone. Aspirin or an anti-inflammatory may ease the pain, as may, in some cases, injecting cortisone around the coccyx.

Referred Pain

Referred pain is pain from another part of your body that may affect your spine. Kidney problems, various infections, menstrual difficulties, and pregnancy are just a few conditions that can result in back pain. Remember Audrey's herniated disk? She first felt pain in her ankle, not her lower back. When a nerve root is irritated, pain radiates elsewhere in the body.

Many women suffer from low-back pain during their menstrual period. Exercising prior to and during your period may alleviate or mitigate that pain. One of the easiest exercises is to lie on your back, bring your knees to your chest, put your arms around your knees, and rock back and forth. This relieves tension on both the lower back and abdominals.

With persistent pain or increasingly severe pain, consult a doctor to rule out such serious health conditions as kidney disease, bowel or bladder problems, gynecological problems, prostate problems, neurological disorders, or tumors. Remember to consult a physician immediately if your back pain interferes with sleep or if any of the following predominate: leg weakness, loss of bladder or bowel control, abdominal pain, or a history of cancer. Severe pain may be an indication of a more serious problem and should not be taken lightly.

Certainly, if you suffer from back pain, more than likely you have experienced one or more of these conditions throughout your lifetime. Fortunately, many of these conditions can either be avoided or regulated by preventive measures, such as learning how to sit or lift. If prevention is what it takes to straighten out your backbone, consider yourself lucky. In the next chapter we take a look at degenerative disorders, or the inevitable aging process that creates havoc for joints, muscles, and cartilage. Mother Nature is not always kind to the degenerative spine.

Chapter 3

ARTHRITIC AND RHEUMATIC CONDITIONS

Helen sat across from me, shuffling a deck of cards. A tall, elegant, woman in her seventies, it seemed incomprehensible that she had suffered nearly four decades from an array of degenerative back problems. Widowed in her fifties, Helen had remained active in politics, community affairs, and the arts until she became housebound with back pain.

Helen came from a family in which everyone was excessively tall, especially the women. All of her sisters had back problems, and all suffered in silence with their pain. Helen's back problems worsened with age. Never an avid sports fan, Helen had neither exercised nor practiced sports. By the tender age of thirty-five, Helen had already been diagnosed with osteoarthritis in her back. She was told nothing could be done about it. Not one to complain, she plunged through her daily activities, worked, and raised a family.

Her back continued to ache constantly, and at the encouragement of her grown children she began an exercise program for it. It didn't help. Still in pain, she visited a rheumatologist who confirmed ankylosing spondylitis. The doctor informed Helen that her spine looked like swiss cheese and that some of the pain was caused by spinal stenosis, a narrowing of the spinal canal. She walked, took her medicine, played with her grandchildren, and suffered in silence. By the time Helen was in her late seventies, the pain was intolerable. She went to a pain clinic, and for nearly two years she suffered with various injections into the spine. Sometimes the injections helped with short-term relief, but after two years with little change in her condition, she had had enough. She wasn't surprised that osteoporosis, an unfortunate condition of bone mass deterioration in aging women, had long since added to the fragility of her spine.

The activities that we take for granted—getting out of bed, walking—riddled Helen with pain. This vital community activist became a recluse. She needed help to get down the stairs, in and out of the car, and into her own house. She reasoned that this was no way to live. Helen had never been a weak or sickly individual, yet pain plagued her days and nights. She decided to give it one more chance before shriveling up in a chair. She returned to an orthopedic surgeon, who again X-rayed Helen's spine. He confirmed Helen's fears: Not much could be done at her age to reverse the degenerative process already in full force. He felt sure that her spine might collapse if they performed surgery. Undeterred, Helen decided surgery was her last option. A year after working with the orthopedist, Helen was operated on. The surgery, a laminectomy fusing the bones together, was considered a great success at her age. But because of the fragility of Helen's spine, the doctor could not implant metal screws to hold the spine in place. Helen tolerated the surgery and, from a medical viewpoint, recovered quickly. The pain, however, did not completely dissipate.

Today Helen walks with a walker, and her determination keeps her going.

"I have bad spells, and oddly enough, the weather seems to affect my arthritis. Some days are better than others, but I intend to get rid of this walker and move on with my life."

Helen's problem is severe, yet Helen says that in retrospect, if doctors had known then what they know today about arthritic and rheumatic conditions affecting the spine, she might not be in the situation she is in today.

"No one mentioned exercise forty years ago, and osteoporosis was still lurking in the Dark Ages. My family's back problems were relegated to long backs and height, not familial degenerative back causes," she recalls.

THE AGING SPINE

A constellation of degenerative changes plague the aging spine. When you hear the term *degenerative arthritic and rheumatic conditions*, you normally think of the fingers, knees, or hands. Although arthritic and rheumatic conditions may not originate in the lumbar region, they can affect the back.

Most of us pay little attention to aching joints. Why should we? We assume the pain will disappear. When the pain doesn't dissipate, we become concerned and go to the doctor in search of answers. We hear a tongue-twister of a diagnosis—say, osteoarthritis, or maybe ankylosing spondylitis, fibromyalgia or rheumatoid arthritis—a new vocabulary of wear and tear and mysterious anatomical alterations. Like all changes that occur within one's body or throughout one's life, understanding and education help relieve the uncertainty that shrouds change. To that end, we'll explore the most common types of rheumatic and arthritic conditions first: osteoarthritis, rheumatoid arthritis, and spondyloarthropathies. Many of these conditions, as mentioned earlier, do not begin in the spine but may ultimately travel to the lumbar region.

OSTEOARTHRITIS

Seventy-year-old Sheila Latasa had hip replacement surgery last May. Three months later, her husband Phil also had hip surgery. The "hip-hip-hooray" culprit, as the Latasas refer to their condition, was osteoarthritis.

Eighty percent of the population over age fifty-five has osteoarthritis, the loss of protective cartilage that results in abnormalities surrounding the bone. Osteoarthritis strikes in two forms: primary, the most common, progressive type that sets in around age forty-five, and the secondary form resulting from a trauma or injury. Traditionally, the variable stiffness, crackling, and joint swelling are managed through exercise, weight control, and anti-inflammatory drugs.

Osteoarthritis also affects the spine, and it can be painful at any age. The result of any arthritis are painful joints, but each condition has particular symptoms. Helen, like the Latasas for example, suffers from osteoarthritis, often called *degenerative arthritis*, which is one of the most common ailments. Approximately forty million Americans have osteoarthritis, and among Americans over age sixty-five, one in eight has symptomatic osteoarthritis. The condition commonly affects the small joints in the hands, the hip, the knee, and the spine.

Rebuilding damaged cartilage has long been the holy grail of orthopedics and rheumatology. The word *arthritis* means "joint irritation." Joint irritation is a relatively common inflammatory disease of the spine and can result in alterations in the cartilage around the bony tissues and joints. But hope may be on the homeopathic horizon.

Amal Das, Jr., M.D., an orthopedic surgeon specializing in hip and knee replacement in Hendersonville, North Carolina, was searching for a "biological alternative" to joint replacement when he stumbled across glucosamine and chondroitin in a number of European medical reviews. The magnetic sulfate combination—glucosamine, a building block and key element that nourishes cartilage, and chondroitin, which inhibits enzyme breakdown of cartilage—is produced naturally in the body. The non-toxic supplements have no apparent side effects. Dr. Das, who is conducting the only clinical study in the United States, gives 1,500 milligrams of glucosamine and 1,200 milligrams of chondroitin in a capsule called Cosamin to patients with moderate osteoarthritis. Veterinarians have been giving this supplement to dogs with arthritic conditions for several years.

The sulfate combination isn't cheap, however. A month's supply hovers around $60. And because it's labeled an alternative supplement, it is not FDA regulated or approved. Also, the supplements sold in the health food stores do not have enough milligrams to really combat the condition.

Causes

When your body's shock absorber, or cartilage, wears out or is injured, the result is the degeneration of the cartilage cap joint surface at the end of the bones. Bone then crunches against bone. This is not an overnight process, but when it does occur, you can feel or hear the joint as it grates. Bone spurs, or osteophytes, may develop, which are pouches of bone at the edge of the joints in the spine, and these osteophytes can press on the nerves, producing a miserable amount of back pain. The cause of osteoarthritis is categorized as either idiopathic or primary. Idiopathic indicates that the origin is unknown. Primary osteoarthritis points to an infection, injury, disease, or a congenital disorder.

Symptoms

The classic symptom of osteoarthritis is pain without activity upon waking. The pain subsides with movement and intensifies in damp weather. Sitting for a prolonged period of time causes the spine to hurt.

Researchers have zeroed in on a protein called type II pro-collagen. This protein forms coils that intertwine in partners of three to build the cartilage that protects bone ends and reduce friction. Due to a breakdown in the gene that instructs the cartilage cells to manufacture collagen, the triple coils in the arthritis sufferers begin to unravel after twenty or thirty years. The result is a breakdown of the protective cartilage cushion, often at a younger age than the usual onset of osteoarthritis.

Traditional Treatment of Osteoarthritis

Your doctor will take an X ray. If only wear and tear of the bone shows up, and nothing else, osteoarthritis spondylitis may be the prime suspect.

Early on, osteoarthritis spondylitis can be managed with rest; regular, gentle exercise; good muscle tone; and proper weight balance. Analgesic medication and nonsteroidal anti-inflammatory drugs (NSAIDs) are often prescribed.

RHEUMATOID ARTHRITIS

This form of arthritis, often called "crippling arthritis," usually afflicts the knee, hip, hand, neck, and wrist joints, but it can also homestead in the lumbar spine. It most often occurs in the fourth and fifth decade of life; the onset of rheumatoid arthritis after the age of sixty-five is rare. A systemic disease, affecting the body as a whole and inflicting joint deformity, it is more common in women than in men. No one knows the cause of rheumatoid arthritis, although many scientists believe a genetic predisposition may trigger its onset.

With rheumatoid arthritis, the immune system attacks the joints as if they were an enemy. The response is a chain reaction of the autoimmune system. As the synovial joints become inflamed, the swelling weakens whatever gets in their path. Ligaments weaken and muscles move out of alignment. It's all out war on the body. Rheumatoid arthritis can progressively worsen, stay the same, then attack again with a vengeance.

Symptoms

The first symptom of rheumatoid arthritis is malaise and fatigue, plus morning tenderness and prolonged stiffness of the joints, particularly in the hands and feet. At this stage, white blood cells are massing and the synovial joints, located throughout the body, begin to fill with new blood vessels. Something has to give. In response to an attack, the cells forming the synovial membrane begin to proliferate. As symptoms intensify, drug therapy is used to prevent irreversible cartilage loss or deformity. If joint swelling worsens, the inflammation process proceeds to the cartilage, tendons, and bone. In the final stages, overgrowth of cartilage and destruction of the bone throw ligaments out of position. Unfortunately, at this point, the battle is lost; destruction at this late stage is irreversible.

Treatment of Rheumatoid Arthritis

Remain active. Do not go to bed, as this only results in weakening muscles. Exercise for at least twenty minutes a day to help build muscle strength. Work with your rheumatologist and educate yourself about this disease. Anti-inflammatory drugs reduce pain, NSAIDs being the initial choice of drugs to help reduce swelling and pain in the joints. If NSAIDs do not work, you may be given cortisone to reduce inflammation. Because cortisone produces possible side effects, such as fluid retention, edema, or loss of calcium from the bones, the severity of rheumatoid arthritis compared to the long term effects must be carefully balanced.

Stages of Rheumatoid Arthritis

In its early stages, rheumatoid arthritis generally presents no symptoms. However, deep in the synovial joints specialized types of white blood cells are forming. Once these cells attach to the joint lining, they turn like an enemy on the white blood cells that make antibodies that attack the joint.

When fluid is taken from the synovial joints and tested, a high white count points to rheumatoid arthritis. Subsequently, a blood test reveals a "rheumatoid factor" antibody found in 80 percent of sufferers. Another feature of rheumatoid arthritis is the rheumatoid nodule, a painless lump you can feel under the skin.

DETERIORATING FACET JOINTS

The unrelenting pain in her lower back kept Sandra awake. She found some relief by sleeping on the couch, adjusting her lower back to wedge between the crack of the cushions. The pain plagued her for days. In the past, her back problems had been minimal and relieved by an osteopath, who could provide her with immediate results. But now, upon Sandra's fourth visit to the osteopath with no change in her condition, she was sent to an orthopedic surgeon, who took X rays. Sandra learned that she had a degenerating disk. The intense pain dominating her life was caused by the facets rubbing up against each other. Although the pain came on suddenly, and may have resulted from lifting something, the degenerative condition had taken time to develop.

Other mitigating factors may have affected Sandra's facet joints. She had developed asthma in her thirties and took prednisone to control it. Later her thyroid gland was removed, due to radiation treatment she'd been given as a child for enlarged thymus glands. Now, at only forty-five, Sandra was diagnosed with osteoporosis and degenerative hip problems. To look at her beautiful face directing a schoolyard full of preschool children, one would never have known how much back pain she suffered.

Both Sandra and her doctor felt surgery was not the best option for her facet pain. Together with a physical therapist, they came up with an exercise plan to strengthen Sandra's back and ease some of the pain. Lifting anything, even preschool children, was deemed out of the question.

Facet joint problems can begin quite painlessly. Irritation of facet joints may, however, be the predominant cause of low back pain. Injury to facet joints leads to irregular bone formation in the area, which occurred in Sandra's case. Joints may become loose, dislocate, or degenerate. Lifting, twisting, and compression can all result in injury to joints.

ANKYLOSING SPONDYLITIS

Ankylosing spondylitis is a chronic rheumatic inflammatory disorder of unknown cause that primarily involves the spine. It is sometimes referred to as Marie Strumpell disease.

"Ankylosing" means stiffening, "spondy" means spine, and "itis" means inflammation. Typically, ankylosing spondylitis begins at the base of the spine and progresses up the spinal column over a period of years. It involves the sacroiliac joints and is three times more prevalent in men than in women. It's often overlooked in women.

In women with ankylosing spondylitis, pelvic pain may be present and is sometimes misdiagnosed as PID, pelvic inflammatory disease. The two disorders should not be confused. With PID, the classic symptoms are low abdominal pain, vaginal discharge, nausea, vomiting, and menstrual irregularities. A good, skilled physician should be able to rule out PID. Ankylosing spondylitis ultimately reveals loss in the lumbar lordosis with total mild restriction. This is not a symptom of PID.

Ankylosing spondylitis is considered the prototype of a group of diseases known as the seronegative spondyloarthropathies, so named because the rheumatoid factor, present in rheumotoid arthritis, is usually not present in the serum of an affected person, and because of the predilection for spinal involvement. It seems to appear in the third or fourth decade of life, with the onset uncommon after age forty.

Symptoms

Ankylosing spondylitis predominately affects young adults, who experience an insidious onset of morning stiffness and low back pain. The pain can be achy or sharp, and may settle in the pelvis, buttocks, or hips. The pain, caused by severe inflammation of the spinal joints, is unrelieved by rest and improved with exercise. When ankylosing spondylitis ascends to the thoracic region, chest constriction can cause respiratory or breathing problems. Smoking is particularly bad for your health in this case.

Discovery

In 1973, an association was discovered between ankylosing spondylitis and HLA-B27, a gene that is highly associated with rheumatoid diseases. The blood test yielding this information, although an important breakthrough, is not always reliable. It does, however, provide the first clue to a relationship between the major immune compatibility complex and disease. Although HLA-B27 is present in the majority of patients with ankylosing spondylitis, most persons who are positive for HLA-B27 do not have the disease.

Ankylosing spondylitis may also be associated with heredity and immunosusceptibility.

Controlling Ankylosing Spondylitis

Swimming and extension exercises are highly recommended, but good posture is still the most valuable therapeutic intervention for ankylosing spondylitis. Joint pain can be relieved by taking NSAIDs. There is no known treatment, but excellent control can be attained. The goal is to relieve pain, and the outlook is good. Ankylosing spondylitis does not usually disrupt lifestyles, but it usually does cause some spinal deformity.

Reiter's Syndrome

Reiter's syndrome is rare and found mostly in young men. It may be associated with sexual exposure without the development of any known venereal disease or with bacterial infections of the intestine. It may show up in susceptible individuals with some infectious agents, such as chlamydia.

Reiter's syndrome is sometimes called:

- Blennorrheal idiopathic arthritis

- Arthritis urethritica

- Venereal arthritis

- Conjunctivourethrosynovial syndrome

- Polyarthritis enterica

Symptoms

Classic symptoms of Reiter's syndrome include joint inflammation; red eyes, or conjunctivitis; and urethritis, which results in pain and burning upon urination. Blood may be apparent in the urine. In later stages, inflammation of the prostate gland or seminal vesicles may occur. Skin eruptions involving the mouth, palms, soles of the feet, and sometime the genitalia occur. They initially resemble small blisters, which become reddish. They cause little pain and disappear quickly. Sometimes the passage leading from the kidneys to the bladder becomes obstructed, causing urethritis. Arthritis usually appears, affecting more joints. Heel pain caused by inflammation of the Achilles tendon is common. These symptoms usually appear over time, and the disease may not be apparent. Reiter's syndrome often coexists with spondylitis.

Treatment of Reiter's Syndrome

Anti-inflammatory drugs such as aspirin, indomethacin, or phenylbutazone usually provide relief. In severe cases, immunosuppressants are given to relieve symptoms. Physical therapy is encouraged during the recovery from the aspect of this condition.

FIBROMYALGIA

Fibromyalgia, commonly called fibrositis, myofibrositis, and fibromyositis, is a syndrome characterized by chronic and widespread musculoskeletal pain throughout much of the body. It affects the muscles and fibrous connective tissue. It does not involve joints as does osteoarthritis or rheumatoid arthritis. Neither the cause nor a cure is known for fibromyalgia.

Symptoms

Fibromyalgia is not life threatening and does not cause deformity, but is commonly misunderstood or diagnosed incorrectly. Believed to be one of the most prevalent rheumatoid disorders, it occurs in approximately 5 percent of the population. Historically, fibromyalgia has been poorly understood and is often referred to as "psychogenic rheumatism." Some physicians feel it is an emotional illness. The major symptoms are fatigue and widespread pain throughout the body. Pain may begin in the neck and shoulders or in the lower back and then spreads. The pain is difficult to describe, although people have referred to it variously as aching, burning, gnawing, and radiating. "Hurting all over" may be a common complaint. Fatigue may be profound. Stiffness in the muscle tissue, especially in the morning, can make it difficult to get out of bed, and the sufferer is tired upon rising. A good night's sleep is unheard of.

Fibrositis is one of the most misunderstood and mistreated disorders in the rheumatic-disease family, even though it affects three million people, the majority of whom are women, who will experience the first symptoms between the ages of twenty and fifty.

Individuals who have fibrositis come to the physician frustrated by the lack of adequate explanation for their symptoms. The pain can be so disabling that sufferers often adhere to a litany of tests with negative results and spend time and money in search of a doctor who will understand their bouts of chronic pain. Sometimes fibrositis exists with another disorder, such as lupus. But many times fibrositis just suddenly appears, like a crushing pain from an accident, and exists without any other medical disorder. Painful points in the back occur in the neck, upper spine, and the upper gluteal or buttocks area.

Treatment of Fibromyalgia

There are few medical treatments for fibromyalgia. Most important, establish a good rapport with your rheumatologist. He or she will take a history and examine the tender points. Since laboratory tests seldom yield results, they should be minimized. A team approach is best for dealing with this painful syndrome. If medication is required, your physician will manage it, as well as coordinate the team effort. Medication is usual in some cases of fibrositis, but not in others. Sometimes NSAIDs or non-narcotic analgesics, such as acetaminophen, may be helpful. Corticosteroids and immunosuppresive drugs or sedatives should be avoided.

In the best possible setting, a physical therapist should help design a home program to aid in pain-reducing techniques and to help stretch tight muscles. Home modalities, such as applying heat and ice, should be discussed. Active exercise is imperative, due to the weakened muscle condition. This can be walking, bicycling, or swimming. Exercise should start slowly and build gradually in duration, according to how much pain can be tolerated.

Because fibrositis can be isolating—one minute you're well; the next your life becomes a debilitating circuit of pain, fatigue, and absence from work—it is important to find a support group. Refer to the appendix for further information on support groups or newsletters on fibrositis.

Polymyalgia Rheumatica

Polymyalgia rheumatica is a chronic episodic inflammatory disease of the large arteries that usually develops in people late in life. It translates as a disorder of many muscle aches of a rheumatic nature and is of unknown cause. Polymyalgia rheumatica has no pathological features attached to it.

Symptoms

Polymyalgia rheumatica typically afflicts women who have been healthy and then become suddenly ill. It primarily affects the muscles, and it is characterized by pain and stiffness of the back, shoulder, neck, and pelvic area. Commonly, the pain begins in the neck and upper arms and radiates toward the elbow. Muscle strength is normal.

The pain tends to be most severe upon arising in the morning. Pain may ease during the day, then increase in the evening. There may be a throbbing headache with this condition, with pain experienced all over. It is not a rare disorder, and there is speculation that polymyalgia rheumatica may be an autoimmune condition. Prednisone is commonly prescribed for pain relief.

While many of the rheumatoid and arthritic conditions affect the general aging population, several, as you have read, strike women more than men. In the following chapter we look at other conditions—some terrifying, like osteoporosis, and others joyful, such as pregnancy—that are particular to women's backs.

Chapter 4

WOMEN'S BACK CONDITIONS

"Age has been unkind to women," grumbled seventy-five-year-old Erma, as the doctor diagnosed a fractured hip. Spry in spirit, frail in body, this was her second trip to the doctor in less than two years. The first time her wrist just snapped during a yoga class for seniors. She'd never broken a bone in her life. Fifteen months later, she lost her balance lifting an empty garbage pail, and this incident resulted in a fractured hip, back pain, and surgery. Erma later learned that she is one of the twenty-four million Americans suffering from osteoporosis.

While osteoporosis is perhaps the most common and severe ailment to plague a woman's body, several other conditions also affect the female spine. Scoliosis, a lateral curve of the spine, and kyphosis, an excessive forward curvature near the shoulders, also create pain and problems. There's probably not a grown woman today who doesn't remember her mother warning her to stand up straight and stick her rump in, otherwise she'd be swayback. Conditions such as pregnancy and child rearing also have an effect on the normal healthy female spine. While we have little control over the onset of osteoporosis or back pain during pregnancy, we do have a modicum of control in our choice of fashionable cosmetic apparatus, such as shoes. Yes, shoes. High heels might be great for creating shapely legs, but they pitch your posture forward, wreaking havoc on the spine. I have no proof, of course, but I suspect high heels were designed by a man, not a woman.

So if you're slender, contemplating pregnancy, have a daughter, are nearing menopause, or simply blowing out one more birthday candle, read on.

OSTEOPOROSIS

Osteoporosis is commonly called a woman's disease. Literally meaning "porous bones," it's a condition that weakens the bones, usually in the spine, hip, and ribs. Bones that were once strong gradually become fragile and prone to fractures. Women are four more times likely to develop osteoporosis than are men.

We've all seen that little old lady—stooped, frail, and bowed because her spine was deformed. We might turn away, too polite to stare. We shake our heads and curse old age, but we think we will never end up like this, in the advanced stages of osteoporosis.

For decades doctors thought of osteoporosis as merely part of the natural aging process for women. Unfortunately, this attitude allowed many practitioners to trivialize the disease. The rationale behind this attitude was if osteoporosis was inevitable, then little could be done about it short of sympathy and a pill. Not much help to the frail woman stooped over in pain.

Today, many leading specialists feel that osteoporosis is a preventable disease, not an inevitable curse of the aging process. Although osteoporosis leads to more than 1.3 million fractures yearly and the National Osteoporosis Foundation estimates that the disease costs us between $7 billion and $10 billion a year, with a $30 billion price tag looming into the next century, prevention is what will keep osteoporosis under control.

What Happens with Osteoporosis

The biological function of the bone is affected with osteoporosis. There is a decrease in normal bone, creating a susceptibility to fractures such as Erma's. The fractures, called fragility fractures, are sometimes painless, other times not.

Loss of bone tissue occurs gradually and without pain. A fracture is the first indication of this condition. Women, such as Helen in chapter 3, who suffered for years with osteoporosis, never knew they had it until an X ray confirmed a broken bone that occurred without an obvious injury. Today doctors can measure the amount of bone in the body with a technique called bone densitometry. Even the smallest loss of bone can be detected. According to the *Osteoporosis Handbook*, by Dr. Sydney Lou Bonnick, a woman is at risk for a fracture when she loses approximately 20 percent of her bone mass. In the United States, more than a million fractures occur from osteoporosis yearly. Of these million, 500,000 are spinal fractures. A third of American women over the age of sixty-five will eventually have a spinal fracture.

A spinal fracture usually occurs without any noticeable injury. The weak bone will break during an ordinary activity, such as picking up a newspaper. But if several vertebrae fracture, the spinal column can collapse on itself. These are called compression fractures, because the vertebral body compresses. The pain caused by this type of spinal fracture can debilitate a woman for several weeks. Sitting up is painful, sleeping is painful, and relief may be up to six months away. With this type of fracture, loss of height and severe curvature of the spine result.

With each impending fracture, loss of height results.

Causes

Although the cause of osteporosis is unknown, many factors contribute to this condition. Numerous studies suggest that bone loss from the spine begins in a woman's forties. Virtually half of all women at age sixty-five, and all women by the age of eighty-five, have endured enough bone loss to risk fractures. Building strong bones, especially before age of thirty, can be the best defense against developing osteoporosis. A healthy lifestyle is critical to keeping bones strong.

Bone Mass. Your bone mass is determined by how much bone you manufactured as a young adult, or peak bone mass. We inherit our ability to make bone mass from our parents. Eighty percent of peak bone mass is most likely determined genetically. The remaining bone mass is determined by nutrition, exercise, illness, estrogen, smoking, and alcohol consumption.

Early Menopause. Women lose bone tissue rapidly after menopause due to a decline in estrogen, a hormone produced in the ovaries that has a protective effect on bone. Bone loss from estrogen deficiency can increase as much as 7 percent a year. During the duration of regular menstrual cycles, women maintain a healthy level of estrogen from puberty to menopause. But early menopause or surgically induced menopause, where the ovaries are removed, increases a woman's chances of developing osteoporosis. Women who have intermittent cycles, or conditions such as anorexia or bulimia, may also be at risk.

While estrogen replacement is considered controversial and risky by many, it plays an effective role in the possible prevention of osteoporosis. Both estrogen and alendronate (a class of drug called *bisphosphonates*) are approved by the FDA for the prevention of osteoporosis. Experts concur that hormone replacement therapy is a viable option for women who are at high risk for osteoporosis, especially if the ovaries have been removed prior to age fifty. Women who have experienced natural menopause but have multiple osteoporosis risk, such as early menopause, a family member with osteoporosis, or are below normal bone mass on a bone density test, are good candidates for HRT. Depending on your medical history, estrogen replacement may have links to cancer, particularly of uterine and breast cancer. The risk of uterine cancer may be offset by adding another hormone, progesterone, to the estrogen therapy. Estrogen replacement comes in the form of pills, injections, vaginal creams, gels, pellets, and patches. While all women experience bone mass loss with age, not everyone opts for the same solution. The long-term use of HRT may have an increased breast cancer factor associated with it, so discuss all pros and cons of estrogen replacement with your doctor.

Age. The longer you live, the higher your chances are for developing osteoporosis. Bone mass gradually declines with age. The older you become, the greater the loss of bone. Although we all lose bone tissue as we age, a woman with osteoporosis has an excessive loss of bone tissue that is not associated with the normal aging process.

Body Type. Slight, small-framed women are at greater risk. Petite women have less bone to lose than do larger-boned women. Genetically, Asian, Caucasian, and Hispanic women tend to be at greater risk than African-American women. Reasons for this are unknown.

Calcium and Diet. We already know that early menopause increases a woman's osteoporosis risk. Recent studies, though, also link an inadequate calcium diet in the early decades of life to osteoporosis. Bone formation and maintenance require a calcium-rich diet; calcium is the most important mineral found in the bone. But since the body does not manufacture calcium, we must consume it. Calcium-rich foods—milk, dairy products, broccoli, and canned salmon or sardines are the best source of calcium. More and more women are also adding soy products to their diet in the form of tofu, soy powder, and soy milk, to name a few. For those who cannot get enough calcium in their diet, calcium supplements are recommended. Some experts feel that taking dietary calcium is the simplest way to prevent osteoporosis, regardless of your age.

How much calcium is enough? Postmenopausal women need to take more calcium than younger women do. Pregnancy requires a significant increase in calcium for fetal growth and lactation. If a pregnant woman does not consume enough calcium, the calcium in her bones will deplete in her body's attempt to satisfy the baby's nutritional needs.

Exercise. Inactivity plays an important role in the onset of osteoporosis. Exercise prevents bone loss, and not just any exercise. While swimming is not a weight bearing exercise, walking is. Recent studies show that women who do fifteen to twenty minutes of weight-bearing exercise three to five times a week cut their risk of osteoporosis in half. Some studies have shown a reversal of bone mass loss through twenty minutes of weight-bearing exercise daily. You do not have to lift weights. You can play tennis, bicycle, walk, or jog. You can also sit in the house and ride a stationary bicycle or incorporate 3- to 5-pound weights in your routine. Remember, the sports that cause muscles to work against the force of gravity are the best prevention against bone loss.

Susceptibility. Many medications have a debilitating effect on bones. Thyroid hormone and corticosteroids like prednisone are the most common culprits implicated in osteoporosis. Remember Sandra in chapter 3? She took prednisone, which she considered a dreadful drug, for a thyroid gland deficiency. The onset of her osteoporosis in her mid-forties had a suspected link to prednisone. So do not stop taking medications, but do discuss their side effects with your physician.

While the statistics on osteoporosis may sound grim, research on osteoporosis has made great strides. No one today will give you a pat on the back, send you home, and cluck about the aging process. It might be late in the game for some of us to start prevention, but it's not too late to get started educating and nourishing your children. With a knowledge of osteoporosis, you can help your children develop healthy bone mass. New drugs and tests are currently on the horizon to prevent osteoporosis. Ask your doctor for further information on these.

With the advent of HMOs, doctors often have little time to spend administering information. Take it upon yourself to do a bit of medical sleuthing. There are numerous books available, or if you have access to a computer, you'll find a wealth of information on the Internet.

PREGNANCY

Pregnancy is hardly a disease. For most women it is a joyous occasion. Pregnancy, however, causes a woman's body to undergo both hormonal and structural changes. And many of these changes can play a role in back pain.

As the pregnancy progresses, the uterus enlarges, weight changes, and the center of gravity shifts forward. The added weight, which increases the normal lumbar curve and the cervical curve, causes a pregnant woman to lean back. This is one reason for low back pain. Second, pregnancy releases the hormone relaxin to loosen the pelvic ligaments in preparation for delivery. This allows the pelvis to stretch for the passage of the baby's head during delivery. Unfortunately, the hormone causes *all* the joints and ligaments in the body to become elastic and unstable.

Low back pain during delivery, also called back labor, is not uncommon. While there is no solution to this excruciating pain, it does pass. No one knows why some women experience low back pain during labor, while others do not. Massage may help, or changing positions during labor. Squatting pulls the center of gravity downward, and some women report temporary relief with this position. Epidural injections during delivery may cause back pain for some time after delivery.

Your doctor may suggest exercise for back pain during pregnancy. Walking, swimming, and prenatal yoga are frequently recommended. Certain stretching exercises should, however, be avoided. Ask your doctor for more specific information.

Postpartum Back Blues

Everyone loves a pregnant woman; she's pampered and praised. Then the baby arrives. Attention shifts to the new arrival, and Mom no longer receives pampering or much help. A first-time mom, who is so busy taking care of a new infant, often ignores her own needs.

But after your baby's birth, a word of caution: *Take care of yourself and your back*.

Abdominal muscles, weak from being stretched during pregnancy, do not support the back adequately and must be strengthened over time. Motherhood is very demanding on the back. Stooping over cribs, picking up infant car seats, and loading down your body with baby paraphernalia all take their toll. The stress of new mothering, weakened abdominal muscles, and constant bending and lifting are sufficient reasons for your back to revolt.

When I first began breast-feeding my daughter I envisioned myself the embodiment of the 1905 Picasso painting of *mère et enfant*—the beautiful woman elegantly breast-feeding her contented baby. But after a week of nursing a new baby, it was obvious that Picasso may have had an eye for women but knew nothing of breast-feeding, even on canvas.

Breast-feeding can be hard on your back, as you hunch over while feeding your infant. Feeding a hungry baby takes patience and good positioning. Tensing at the neck, shoulders, and back can all translate into back pain that persists even when you've finished feeding the baby. Despite my luck in having a lactation consultant to coach me, it still took some time for me to relearn proper feeding techniques to relieve the pain in my own neck and back.

It is important not to slump or round your shoulders when breast-feeding. You have enough stress with bringing a new baby home without having an aching back during feeding time. To avoid back problems, sit in a comfortable chair and support your baby with a pillow. Bring the baby to the breast, not your breast to the baby. Try to maintain good posture during breast-feeding. Ask your doctor or nurse practitioner for common sense breast-feeding positions, or read one of the many pamphlets or books on breast-feeding for suggested postures.

Even if you choose not to breast-feed, looking down at your baby while holding a bottle stresses the base of the neck. Gently tilt your head back and forth or to the side to exercise the neck muscles.

Carrying. Carrying an infant, particularly a large one, pulls your body forward. This results in rounded shoulders and upper back pain. If you hold your baby on one side of your body, your muscles on that side compensate leaning in that direction. Switch sides and switch positions. Avoid carrying your baby on one hip; it throws your posture and back out of alignment. Try to keep your baby off the hip and more toward the center of your body. Always contract your stomach muscles when lifting an infant.

Lifting. Think about how many times in your child's life you will lift him or her out of the crib—a lot. And, if you bend over and over without thinking about your back, it will eventually revolt. Again, tighten your stomach muscles and bend your knees a bit. Most cribs have a side that you can release and pull down. Get in the practice of lowering this side to retrieve your infant so that you don't have to reach over the top of the crib and then bend down. This not only stresses your lower back, but your upper back as well. Have your toddler stand up in the crib before lifting him or her. When lifting a child off the floor, bend your knees and squat a little.

Bathing and the Back. As my daughter got older, I noticed that my back bothered me every time I bathed her. Bending over a bathtub is like bending over a vacuum cleaner, one does it unconsciously, bet seldom correctly. Do not stand up and bend over the bathtub to bathe your child. Get on your knees or sit on a stool. Again, bend your knees and tighten your stomach muscles when lifting little ones out of the tub. As children get older, take their hands and help them climb over the tub. Never let a young child get out of the tub without help or leave a child unattended in the bath water, no matter how much your back hurts.

SCOLIOSIS

Scoliosis, a derivative of the Greek skoliosis, or "curve," refers to a lateral curve of the spine, such as that suffered by literature's Hunchback of Notre Dame.

Scoliosis is a painless bending and twisting of the upper spinal column, which is sometimes progressive and distorts the chest and back. It went unrecognized for centuries until the mid-1960s, when the Scoliosis Research Society was established. Since the sixties, awareness of scoliosis, especially in school-age children, has grown dramatically. Researchers have tracked every nook and cranny of the body to find a logical explanation for scoliosis, with little success. The nature of scoliosis can be either structural or nonstructural. Some causes of nonstructural scoliosis are leg-length discrepancies, postural problems, muscle spasms, and spinal tumors. In a mild case of nonstructural scoliosis, something as simple as using a heel lift to level the sacral base can be beneficial.

Structural scoliosis, on the other hand, is most commonly idiopathic, or of un-known origin. Sometimes structural scoliosis is cased by a birth defect, such as spina bifida, or a severe accident or neuromuscular disorder, such as polio, but 80 percent of the cases have no such etiology. Scoliosis occurs during the growing years at different life stages: Infantile (birth to three years), juvenile (three years to ten years), and adolescent (ten years and up).

Infantile idiopathic scoliosis appears more in male than in female infants and usually disappears without treatment in the first years of life. Infantile scoliosis is a rare condition. In 95 percent of all cases, it improves on its own. For unknown reasons, infantile idiopathic scoliosis occurs far more often in Europe than in the United States.

Juvenile idiopathic scoliosis may develop after age three and prior to puberty. This form does not always correct itself and often increases with time. It requires treatment such as bracing; otherwise, spinal malformation may result.

Adolescent idiopathic scoliosis is by far the most prevalent. It occurs during the growth spurt and is diagnosed when a curve is discovered. The curve may have been present for some time. The younger the child develops a curve, the less favorable the prognosis, due to a longer period of progression. This type, for some unknown reason, strikes females more than males.

Scoliosis is often detected by a doctor or simple screening test at school. In the early stages, there are no obvious symptoms. In the later stages, there is visible body curvature. The spine becomes S-shaped and the shoulders uneven.

Spinal Curves

Scoliotic curves are measured in degrees. Often two people may have the same degree of curve but are treated differently, depending on the age of the individual and age of the bones. Curves are complicated, but to help educate the person with scoliosis, doctors use the Cobb angle of measurement, which measures the amount of spinal rotation. Although doctors have identified nearly a dozen various curve patterns, let's look at the four most common:

• The most prevalent curve is the right thoracic curve, which centers in the chest. This type of curve progresses rapidly, and if not treated will shift the ribs to create a deformity known as a rib hump on the back. If severe, it can squeeze the heart and lungs, creating serious cardiopulmonary problems.

• The thoracolumbar curve begins in the chest area and ends in the lower back. It may twist in either direction, and although less deforming, it creates an asymmetrical torso.

• The lumbar curve presents in the lower back and in most cases shifts to the left. This type of curve causes back pain, particularly in adults, due to the twist in the hips.

• The double major curve is the most prevalent of the S-shape scoliosis curves. The upper part of the curve takes form in the chest area, while the lower part affects the lumbar area. Because the curves offset each other, this type of scoliosis is less deforming. But if left unchecked, it can cause a hump.

Warning Signs

There isn't a parent who doesn't at some time harp at a teenager to stand up straight and quit slumping. One of the first warning signs of scoliosis is poor posture, although side by side, simple poor posture and scoliosis appear much different. In normal but poor posture, the head is in line with the buttocks, and the shoulders and hips are symmetrical. Scoliosis may be suspected if the shoulders and hips are uneven, and the waist is lopsided. Clothes fit improperly—a hem may appear uneven or a pant leg shorter. Pain, especially among teenagers, is not usually a symptom. Adults with advanced scoliosis, however, may experience pain due to subsequent breathing problems or arthritic conditions.

Treatment of Scoliosis

Treatment depends on severity and the child's age, health, and underlying disorders. Today the most widely accepted therapies are bracing and spinal fusion.

Bracing is recommended for growing children with curves greater than 20 or 25 degrees, but less than 40 degrees. The Milwaukee brace, developed in 1945, extends from the chin to the pelvis. More recently developed braces may not include the neck area and are more easily tolerated.

Braces are worn twenty-three hours a day and are prescribed during the growing years to prevent the progression of scoliosis. Sometimes surgery is necessary, in spite of bracing.

When curves are diagnosed later rather than earlier, sometimes spinal fusion surgery is the answer. The surgery can be performed anteriorly or posteriorly. Years ago, patients stayed in bed after surgery, but this is no longer so. Today patients are up and walking after two or three days.

In 1960, the first school program for screening children for scoliosis was instituted. Today such screening is common nationwide. When diagnosed early, scoliosis can usually be completely corrected.

For further resources on scoliosis, check the appendix.

KYPHOSIS

Kyphosis is an abnormal condition of the vertebral column characterized by an excessive forward curve of the thoracic spine at the shoulder blades. The hump that women develop with osteoporosis is kyphosis. It is incorrectly called dowager's hump or widow's hump.

Kyphosis may be caused by rickets or tuberculosis of the spine. In adolescents, however, kyphosis is often self-limiting and undiagnosed. If the curvature progresses, moderate back pain may result.

Conservative treatment of kyphosis calls for spine-stretching exercises and sleeping without a pillow on a hard mattress. A modified brace may also be employed in severe cases.

Although severe kyphosis is less common than scoliosis, it is more serious, especially in young girls. In older people, osteoporosis may be causal in kyphosis.

LORDOSIS

Lordosis is far more common in young girls than in young boys. Lordosis, commonly called swayback, is an exaggeration of the normal lumbar curve of the back. When I was a teenager, my mother used to berate me for standing swayback.

Truly, at thirteen years old, I didn't have a clue what she was talking about. But if you can show your daughter her posture in a mirror and she can see that the curve in her lower back exaggerates, throwing the rest of her structure out of alignment, she might get the picture. Unfortunately, poor posture seems to be a national problem for teenagers; it is certainly the most significant problem affiliated with lordosis.

Vertebral Osteochondritis

Also called juvenile kyphosis and Scheuerman's disease, vertebral osteochondritis is an uncommon condition that primarily affects teenagers, both girls and boys.

Changes at the junction of the vertebrae and disks of the thoracic spine create increased curvature, with pain in the thoracic area. At times, if left unattended, pain may persist and compression of the spinal cord may occur. Treatment usually involves a brace until the patient has stopped growing in order to prevent deformity.

Easy Does It

When back pain is related to quotidian habits, such as wearing high heels, balancing your child on your hip, or toting the diaper bag on your shoulder, there are some simple solutions.

Take off the high heels, and keep them off. Buy a pair of flat shoes for walking. Learn to carry your child in front, while flexing your abdominals. Don't carry more weight than you can manage. Look in the mirror and watch what loading your body down like a camel does to your posture. You're not going across the desert, you're probably just going around the corner to the store.

While we ask ourselves why certain conditions affect a woman's body, we must also feel fortunate, moving as we are into the next century, that so many strides have been made. No, we still don't have the answer for why osteoporosis or scoliosis afflicts women, but we do have many more answers than we did thirty years ago. Prevention may be just a few decades away. Pain, however, lives in the present. If you suffer from pain, or if a loved one is in chronic pain, the next chapter is worth a read.

Chapter 5

WHAT IS PAIN?

What is pain? Ask Bob Tellería, executive director of For Those In Pain, Inc., a nonprofit agency aimed at helping people lessen the difficulty of physical pain, suffering, and disability. The agency offers low-cost advocacy, referrals, education, and emotional support services.

Tellería is personally acquainted with pain. In 1996, he suffered a spinal cord injury when his chair collapsed, and he spent five months wearing a halo supporting his head and spine and a spinal fusion. This has not stopped Bob's determined spirit along with the help of two canes and a wheelchair. He defies the path that many chronic pain patients tread—feeling useless and sorry for themselves. As he is fond of saying, "Any competent person who struggles with significant ongoing pain will from time to time feel like a deer staring at headlights."

Tellería's personal experience with chronic pain was the motivation to found For Those In Pain, Inc. This organization helps people navigate the health-care labyrinth, routine insurance conundrums, legal and family implications, and, most importantly, the personal territory of one's own heart.

In addition to advocacy and referrals, Tellería offers one-on-one counseling, group education, support, and community teaching. No one is turned away from For Those

In Pain due to lack of ability to pay. Tellería's experience has taught him that chronic pain patients are like everyone else—irreducibly valuable. A patient's first call for help results in a thirty or forty minute session. Every patient is treated with respect and with the conviction that the most indispensable key to effective pain management is the person experiencing the pain.

Pain is a warning system to alert us that something is askew in our body. Pain signals are distressing, especially if we can't immediately locate the source. Pain is personal, and what may be trivial pain for one may be unbearable for another. Chronic back pain festers in this unbearable category.

The toll of pain in terms of human suffering is astounding. Economically, you cannot price misery, but statistics indicate just how prevalent pain is felt in our society. According to *The Chronic Pain Control Workbook*, a step-by-step guide to coping with pain, the most chronic of musculoskeletal pains is back pain. Fifteen percent of the adult U.S. population has persistent low back pain at some time in their lives. Five million Americans are partially disabled by back problems, and another two million are so severely disabled they cannot work. Low back pain accounts for ninety-three million workdays lost every year, at a cost of $5 million in health care.

Nevertheless, most back attacks pass within a matter of days or weeks. Back attacks announce themselves unexpectedly, and if treated conservatively, go away without too much interference. (Although anyone who has suffered from a severe back attack will tell you that the excruciating pain seems to go on forever.)

Your doctor may diagnose your back pain as acute or chronic. He or she may be able to locate the reason why your back hurts. A more common scenario, however, is that your practitioner will not be able to determine the causes of your backache.

Unexplained pain frightens a healthy person. In the acute stage, back pain may give way to drawn-out pain or long-term pain. At this juncture in your quest for answers you may run the gamut of doctors, take muscle relaxants, endure physical therapy, and even rest—all to no avail. Pain dominates, ruling everything you do. It inhibits your lifestyle and work patterns. Frustration triggers anger. After months and sometimes years, it is clear that your body will never again be pain free. Relationships nose-dive. Friends beg for a respite from the litany of complaints; your spouse feels put-upon, overwhelmed by the tasks you once did that are now relegated to him or her; sex is painful, if existent; your children retreat from your reptilian mood swings;

and your self-esteem plummets when you realize that the workforce shuns a chronic pain sufferer. Vexed at the painful turn of events ruling your life, you question why, with all our access to modern medical research and technology, you are left to your own mental devices to control the ceaseless pain destroying your life.

PUTTING BACK PAIN IN HISTORICAL PERSPECTIVE

If you view back pain in its historical perspective, you may be able to better understand why managing back pain often falls upon the individuals.

Back pain is mankind's oldest agony. So prestigious is this pain that magazines, such as *Time* and *Smithsonian,* have featured it as the complaint of the year. But despite its notoriety, back pain has resisted inroads to its progress. Instead, we have created more opportunities to injure our back than did our ancestors. Sedentary lifestyle, work-related injury, and longevity all wreak havoc on the spine.

In the old days, people with backaches kept on going; they seldom sought medical help. Today, people seek out doctors for back pain relief, only to find themselves outside the purview of a cure.

Much of spinal medicine is still in its infancy. The first fellowship in spine care occurred in the 1970s. Until then, orthopedists were ignored by fellow neurosurgeons, who at that time performed spine surgery. Certainly chiropractors and acupuncturists have been on the scene for centuries, but their segue into the halls of modern American medicine has not been easy. And in the last forty years, new pain theories have defied the traditional theory of how doctors view pain.

THE PAIN SPECTRUM

Backaches and chronic pain are age-old companions. Because pain is one of the first warning signals of back problems, understanding the types of pain that afflict your back is important.

1. Acute pain is short-term pain. Its purpose is to alert you that something is wrong. It is triggered by the nervous system and may result from an injury or trauma. Acute pain requires immediate attention because of potential tissue damage. When the cause of acute pain is attended to, the pain goes away.

2.   Chronic pain is different. It persists. Your mind as well as your body gets involved. Fiendishly, pain signals keep firing in the nervous system. Chronic pain is unremitting and demoralizing; it can affect your emotional state, self-esteem, and relationships; it can virtually become a way of life, and not a pleasant one. Chronic pain does not respond to the same treatment used for acute pain. It's in a league all its own, and it mystifies even the experts.

3.   Referred pain describes chronic pain that has moved past the initial source of irritation. In other words, it has relocated from the original spot to somewhere else in your body. Characteristics of referred pain may be aching joints or muscles, or muscle spasms.

THE PAIN PATH

The adage "Time heals all wounds" holds absolutely nothing for the person in pain. For the individual in chronic pain, pain is a race against time. For centuries pain has been the subject of study, but only in the last thirty years have illuminating discoveries surfaced about our perception and reaction to pain.

Once regarded as a straightforward mechanism, a simple stimulus-response, pain was thought to be directly relayed to the brain. This specificity theory is still widely accepted. The theory suggests that the intensity of the pain is proportional to the wound or damage. In other words, big injury equals big hurt; small injury equals minor hurt. The obvious conclusion this specificity theory points to is that when you medicate or perform surgery, the pain disappears. But chronic pain does not fall into this category.

In 1965, Dr. Ronald Melzack and Dr. Patrick Wall introduced the "gate theory" to medicine, changing the way many clinicians viewed pain. These Canadian and English investigators speculated that the gates on the bundles of nerve fibers, located on the spinal cord, could either open, to allow pain impulses to pass to the brain, or close off. A significant amount of stimuli, such as rubbing, could excite the nerve cells sensitive to touch and pressure to "close the gate" to the pain sensation. Their study also showed that brain-based pain-control systems were activated when people behaved heroically. Soldiers in battle or sports figures could be badly injured but still finish a game or help those soldiers more severely wounded in battle. Negating a simple cause-and-effect relationship, Melzack and Wall's theory describes a complex communication of pain signals, emotions, and thoughts involving different highways or pathways of pain.

Around the time this controversial gate theory appeared, scientists in Aberdeen, Scotland, and Johns Hopkins University in Baltimore discovered pain-suppressing chemicals in the brain: endorphins or enkephalins, the brain's own natural opiates.

The Chronic Pain Circuit

When you cut yourself, nerve endings called pain receptors pick up the pain and act as cables, transmitting pain information from one bunch of nerve fibers to another, and then to cells in the spinal cord, where the cortex picks up the relayed message. *Ouch!* The message is quick, the pain swift.

But in contrast, chronic pain travels a different highway than acute pain. This pain is dull, aching, or burning. While chronic pain starts on the same path, it deviates in the brain stem and moves toward the hypothalamus, the gland that instructs the pituitary gland to release certain stress hormones, and the limbic structures, where emotions are processed.

As the pain embarks on its round trip from the brain back to the wounded area, the brain releases chemical substances and nerve impulses down the cells in the spinal cord to act against the pain message. The gates close in the spinal cord to ascending messages.

Each cell along the nerve tract contains chemical substances called neurotransmitters that act either as painkillers or pain producers. Endorphins, the body's natural painkiller, have the same powerful effect as a drug such as morphine. Individuals produce different amounts of endorphins, and this may explain why people tolerate pain differently. Endorphins are released by nerves in the brain. They are analgesic chemicals which give the body its natural defense against pain. Without endorphins it would hurt to be alive. Neurotransmitters are compounds that convey information from one nerve cell to the other.

Research continues to shed light on the complex relationship involving the brain, the body, and its interweaving of pain signals. But even with all the research, chronic pain still afflicts millions of Americans and baffles even the most knowledgeable of practitioners.

How to Recognize a Chronic Back Pain Cycle

The chronic pain syndrome typically moves in a cyclical pattern. It may commence with an injury. Your back hurts, and you take it easy. You limit activities and expect the pain to ease. If the pain doesn't dissipate, concern can give way to self-pity. You curtail your activities even more. Frustration and depression set in. Some days are better than others, and when your pain level is tolerable, you may overexert yourself. The pain returns with a vengeance, and you're convinced you cannot live life to its fullest. Chronic pain consumes you.

The Painful Spiral

Once chronic pain controls you, it is easy to zoom into a downward spiral, affecting your health and lifestyle. The less active you become due to pain, the weaker you become. If back pain drags on, you fear doing anything that might incite pain. Sleep is a chore; drugs lull you to sleep and exhaustion saps your mental strength. Depression causes you to withdraw, and ultimately you feel victimized. This spiral is self-perpetuating. It requires understanding, personal involvement, and a pain clinic to help control it.

THE PAIN CLINIC

In *Mastering Pain: A Twelve-Step Program for Coping with Chronic Pain,* Dr. Richard A. Sternbach begins his chapter on chronic pain with a quote from Somerset Maugham: "It's not true that suffering ennobles character. Suffering, for the most part, makes men petty and vindictive. There is absolutely nothing ennobling in the human road map of chronic pain."

Arthur Schuller, internist, psychiatrist, and director of the pain clinic at St. Mary's Spine Center in San Francisco, admits that in all his years of practice he has never seen people enlarged by pain. "There is a callousness toward pain in our society," Schuller notes. "Perhaps it is culturally defined, but as a nation, we do not honor each other's suffering."

American culture prizes overcoming afflictions and getting on with life. We consider the individual in chronic pain a drag, a social pariah. In the age of rocket-science medicine, the person suffering pain expects that technology will magically provide deliverance from the ordeal. It doesn't always happen.

Arthur Schuller's office is the last door that a chronic pain sufferer knocks on. It is the door of desperation, the pain sufferer's landscape of hope.

Chronic pain sufferers come to Schuller after they have been treated by the clinic's osteopath, physical therapist, surgeon, or other outside clinicians. They come to Schuller, the psychological shaman at the bottom of the totem pole, in hopes that he can miraculously exorcise their pain.

Immediately, Schuller defines the partnership involving himself, the pain therapist, and the individual seeking relief. Schuller insists that the relationship between the practitioner and the patient must be built on trust, respect, and honesty. It's a committed partnership, a kind of two-way pact. He doesn't tolerate insult, nor would he ever be the arrow bearing insult. With the committed covenant established, therapy begins.

Schuller proceeds to help the individual determine what exactly is to be achieved in the intense pain clinic and what the degree of commitment to that attainment actually is. Once commitment has been established, the patient learns he's to be his own shaman, and that Schuller will facilitate the finding of his path, but that only the individual can walk it.

For an individual who has spent years in chronic pain, old patterns of behavior may have to be dislodged, the past uprooted. As Schuller's clinic emphasizes a commitment to wellness, sometimes unhealthy patterns have to be buried along the way.

Schuller aggressively prescribes nonnarcotic analgesics to displace the pain. "There is no such thing as a useful, inadequate dose of narcotic," says Schuller. So he tries whatever it takes to obtain relief of pain. Once the pain is eased, Schuller embarks upon a course of action. Since individuals respond differently, the course often has its own detours.

The pain clinic commences with a review of activities and body-management techniques. Many of these techniques may be familiar to the patient in pain. Nevertheless, Schuller pushes these techniques one step further. He stresses the importance of recognizing pain tolerance and not pushing the body beyond its boundary. If an injured back tolerates twenty-minute intervals of sitting, and sitting for thirty minutes means the difference between a good day and a bad day, those extra ten minutes become a fine line between recognizing pain tolerance and abusing it. In the pain clinic, individuals learn how to pay attention to their body limits. If twenty minutes is the maximum tolerance in a chair, then Schuller suggests getting off the seat and onto your feet in eighteen minutes. This lesson in getting up and down teaches the individual to stop using pain as an indicator and to start acting appropriately within the constraints of his or her physical universe.

Once the constraints of the physical universe are well understood, pacing oneself becomes easier. Pacing every hour, something that those who have never experienced chronic pain seldom understand, can make all the difference between a good day and a miserable day. If Monday's walk is a fifteen-minute tour around the block, then Tuesday's shouldn't be an hour sprint across the park. The desire to get better often overlooks the body's physical constraints.

Patients are asked to keep a chart of what ignites their pain. By charting a course, one can see what activities or stressful situations tamper with pain.

Schuller's clinic uses progressive techniques, or mindfulness practices such as relaxation, breathing, and visualization. Some patients respond to these techniques and others don't. Some find a temporary respite from pain or use some of these methods to manage pain. Others don't want to bother with these mindfulness techniques. As Schuller will tell you, if the mind is not ready to accept a method, then surely that method will not help the individual.

But Schuller's patients will tell you that the most meaningful part of the pain clinic is that he is there for them. Compassion and commiseration define an essential component on the road to wellness.

"Being with people is important. While a number of people never conquer chronic pain, quite a few learn to manage their pain," says Schuller.

Participating in life once again may be the measure of success for a chronic pain sufferer. The general success rate for back sufferers returning to work with chronic pain is low; only somewhere between 2 and 4 percent make it back to the workforce. In Schuller's clinic, however, about 45 percent return to work. But Schuller cautions against statistics. Do these individuals stay at work, and if so, for how long? That would be the true measure of success.

Chronic pain is a database of statistics: Going back to work after a battle with chronic pain may have nothing to do with the severity of the injury, but rather the individual's attitude about his or her job; and the longer one is out of work, the less likely it is one will return to the workforce. Moreover, victims of physical and sexual abuse continually show up in the chronic pain cycle. But when it comes to chronic pain, the psychology of one's life patterns cannot be ignored. The mind is a powerful tool. Sometimes unpacking our emotional anguish to move through pain is extremely painful and requires a great deal of courage. Many times we choose to leave the trunks of our pain buried in the past. But according to Schuller, one, however, cannot be successful with minimization or control of chronic pain if wedded in a painful history. Sometimes a new identity emerges in the midst of dealing with chronic pain.

The Painful Truth

Fighting chronic pain is a long-term avocation. It requires the tenacity to educate our society about the pervasiveness of chronic pain, and to understand that all people suffer in the same way, no matter what their status in life might be. We hail as a hero the quarterback or basketball star who blows a disk at the tender age of thirty-two, and whose career is finished. We regret his untimely injury, scan the sports section for details, and mourn his departure from our lives.

But when a trash collector blows a disk, or when a truck driver freighting our food cross-country is plagued by sciatica or degenerative disk problems from hours at the wheel, it's a different story. These men too are unable to return to work. These men too become statistics—but not on the roster of heroic databases. No, these men are scorned. They're just cogs in the chain of worker's compensation benefits. Losers, men without jobs. More tragically, they become isolated human beings wondering what the hell happened to their lives.

Schuller's pain clinic, like the hundreds of pain clinics across this country, is not a miracle place; it is the last stop on a very painful journey. Sometimes tiny miracles do occur, like that miracle of becoming pain free. The more common scenario is the individual who learns to work with pain, to take the responsibility of the demon possessing his or her body, and to manage it. *Cure* is a sacred word in pain clinics, and I don't suggest that a person in pain shouldn't strive for miracles. But until that miracle occurs, a more realistic approach is to understand that the management of pain is the instrument that interrupts the cycle of pain, permitting you to move on with your life positively.

What Constitutes a Pain Clinic

Pain clinics are in vogue; they've shot up all around the country. Clinics range in price and content, from simple centers to extensive upscale clinics in hospitals. The primary approach to pain clinics is to recognize the physical, psychological, and social factors involved in chronic-pain management. Different types of specialists work in pain clinics, applying a variety of methods to approach pain. The best pain clinics teach coping skills and also provide state-of-the-art medical treatment. You may want to consider the following factors about a pain clinic before deciding on one.

While there is no uniform method to certify pain facilities, the Commission on Accreditation of Rehabilitation Facilities (CARF) has developed standards for multi-disciplinary clinics, with the help of the American Pain Society. There are 127 CARF-accredited clinics in the United States. Nearly a thousand nonaccredited facilities call themselves pain clinics but may consist of only one practitioner or practice only one type of therapy. A good pain clinic should have a variety of specialists on staff. Because there is no medical residency program for pain management, ask your specialist about his or her training:

• How much experience does the specialist have in pain management? A specialist may be brilliant in his or her field of medicine, but may be new to the field of pain management.

• What types of treatment are used in the pain-management setting? Are relaxation training and biofeedback, a method in which machines help train patients to control the body's involuntary functions in a mind-over-matter approach, part of the pain program?

• What about guided imagery, a technique used to help with stress reduction by bringing the back sufferer into a more soothing state of mind?

• Is hypnosis available or used in conjunction with other techniques?

• Are acupuncture or acupressure offered as an alternative method of controlling pain? Are clinic personnel amenable to it from outside practitioners?

• Is the specialist associated with a pain clinic or with the American Academy of Pain Medicine?

• How do third-party payers influence your treatment? Does your insurance company dictate what your pain clinic can treat? Is there a limit to the number of treatments or types of drugs your policy covers? Unfortunately, with the vast changes in our health care system, the bottom line is all too often money, and not necessarily the best interests of the pain sufferer.

Who Might Be Part of a Pain Clinic

Specialists you might expect to encounter in a pain clinic include an osteopath, anesthesiologist, orthopedist, chiropractor, neurologist, physiatrist, physical therapist, psychiatrist, psychologist, and social worker. Chances are, more than one specialist will be involved in your case. Because chronic pain can be both physically and psychologically debilitating, a combination of psychological and physiological techniques are often recommended. Check the appendix for a listing of pain clinics and support groups.

EMOTIONS AND CHRONIC PAIN TMS

David Schechter, M.D., was a medical student at NYU when he met John Sarno, author of *Mind Over Back Pain* and *Healing Back Pain*—both departures from traditional methods toward healing back ailments. Sarno focuses on the emotional rather than physical cause of back pain. His diagnosis, known as *tension myositis syndrome* (TMS), involves a circuit that connects the emotions, the brain, the limbic system, which is part of the brain, and the autonomic or involuntary nervous system. People who have TMS often have similar personality charateristics. They tend to be motivated, neat, orderly, judgmental, responsible, self-critical, and perfectionist. Medically, his theories have not gained wide acceptance.

But Schechter, who is director of the sports medicine division of the International Orthopedic Center for Joint Disorders in Los Angeles, says he commonly diagnoses TMS. "No one knows how many back pain sufferers have TMS as their primary cause of pain, especially if a doctor is not thinking of it and a patient is not open to it," says Schechter. "The idea that the mind triggers physical discomfort makes many people uncomfortable. But to treat TMS effectively, one has to think psychologically, not physically, be involved with the cure, and acknowledge the role of tension as a pain culprit. That's not easy when tests cannot diagnose TMS in the same way that an X ray can diagnose a fracture," notes Schechter, who gives monthly TMS seminars to his patients.

Thirty-five year old Anne was one of Schechter's patients. She came to his office after having seen two orthopedic surgeons and extensive physical therapy that proved to be ineffective in curing her back pain. Her MRI scans showed minimal degenerative changes but were otherwise normal. She had decreased flexibility in her hips and back but no neurological findings. Anne was a hard-driving perfectionist, professionally successful, but tense. She suffered tension headaches in the past. Schechter examined her, confirmed a diagnosis of TMS, and gave her educational material on TMS. By the time she attended the seminar, she felt 60 percent better, but questioned the diagnosis despite her improvement. Schechter encouraged her to look inside for emotional issues and to take up some of the physical activities, such as biking and hiking, that she stopped because of her pain. One year and several hikes later, Anne reports a 95 percent improvement over her back pain.

REGAINING CONTROL OF YOUR LIFE

Regaining control of your chronic back pain takes time. To reiterate, control comes through understanding chronic pain. It is important not to isolate yourself and to continually seek information on support groups. Pain management requires an active role. You are the key player.

If there is no medical answer or cure for your back condition, accept your condition. Once you've crossed the bridge of acceptance, you can move on and start to make positive changes.

Discuss your feelings with your family, friends, and a support group. Communicating offers a different perspective on the situation. More important, you learn how others manage and perceive pain, and you realize that you are not alone.

Learn to relax: Stress makes chronic back pain worse. Learn techniques to make you more comfortable. Some people use deep breathing or visualization; others go to their library and check out one of many videos or tapes on relaxation. Check the appendix for a list of books and tapes.

Learn to concentrate on your needs, not what your pain dictates. Take the responsibility for meeting your needs and making them known to others.

Pain may be managed, but until that point, it is often very difficult to tolerate. Whether we are in acute or chronic pain, we traditionally seek the quickest form of relief: the kind that comes in a capsule or pill. The next chapter will examine the drugs prescribed for back problems and how they can mask or help your painful condition.

Chapter 6

A CONSERVATIVE COURSE IN TREATMENT DRUGS

When Ken ruptured his disk a few months ago, his doctor gave him a muscle relaxant and sent him home to rest for a few days. The relaxant masked the pain, but not the problem. When Ken tapered off the drug, the pain resurfaced. He realized that a short course of drug treatment made life tolerable, but that he needed something else to more fully correct the disk problem. This was possible with physical therapy, exercise, and changing his work station.

Matthew, on the other hand, suffered with intense back pain for well over a year. He first hurt his back in a gym. Several months later, during a run, a sharp pain shot down his knee, and numbness settled in his calf. An MRI showed a bulging disk, pressing against nerves, and sciatica. An epidural had him terrified and gave absolutely no relief. While experimenting with different practitioners, Matthew started prescribed drugs.

"I must have tried a dozen different kinds of pills. They overwhelmed me, and left me panic stricken," recalls Matthew.

Tossing the pills, Matthew continued his search to alleviate the pain. He rotated between a neurosurgeon, an orthopedist, a physical therapist, an acupuncturist, and various alternative practitioners. Although he vowed to stay off drugs for his pain, several months after his first experience with antisteriods, Matthew went on a trip and reinjured his back. On the advice of a physical therapist, he went swimming. The next morning he could not get out of bed.

The doctor prescribed Valium. Matthew took them, no questions asked. Feeling like a limp noodle, he switched to a mild anti-inflammatory analgesic, Naprosyn. Once he was able to get back on his feet, he pitched the drugs, and with perseverance and a lot of money, he eventually controlled his back injury through a combination of bodywork techniques that will be touched upon in Part II of this book.

THE TEMPORARY TEMPTATION

The first thing many of us do when in pain is reach for a drug. This is understandable; after all, we have been conditioned as a society to search for the quickest form of relief. But while relief might be just a pill away, be cautiously aware that back pain is not cured by taking drugs. Drugs give only temporary relief. Be careful when taking narcotics for your back problems. They are not a solution.

If you have any questions about the drug you have purchased over the counter or that your doctor has prescribed, by all means, consult your physician or pharmacist. Yes, your local pharmacist is a wonderful source of information when it comes to the pills you swallow. Ask for a brief consultation about the drug:

- What are the side effects?

- Should the drug be taken with food or on an empty stomach?

- What does your pharmacist suggest if you have a reaction?

- How potent is the drug compared with another similar drug?

- Are there foods that should not be taken with a specific drug?

- When should you dispose of the drug?

- Can you have an adverse reaction if combined with other medicine?

- Does your pharmacist have an opinion about the drug you are purchasing?

If the differences between anti-inflammatories (or nonnarcotic analgesics), pain-killers, and muscle relaxants confuse you, perhaps your pharmacist can offer more information on the subject or give you a pamphlet.

Drugs for treatment of backaches generally fall into three categories: anti-inflammatories (or nonnarcotic analgesics), painkillers, and muscle relaxants. New drugs are continually being discovered, and some of the new generation of medicines are not habit forming.

Anti-inflammatories or Nonnarcotic Analgesics

Nonnarcotic analgesics fall into two categories. The first, an acetominophen class of drug such as Tylenol, comprise mild analgesics that work for reducing fever. They are not anti-inflammatories. In other words, they are unable to soothe irritated tissue in conditions such as arthritis, because they have no anti-inflammatory agents. They are, however, effective for mild pain.

In the second category are the nonsteroidal anti-inflammatory drugs commonly referred to as NSAIDs. Aspirin is the best known of these. We tend to take an aspirin for all sorts of common ailments, including fever, but aspirin has very effective anti-inflammatory properties. Ibuprofen, Advil, Nuprin, and Motrin are a few of the brand names sold over the counter.

The theory is that NSAIDs work to reduce the tissue concentrations of chemicals involved in the production of inflammation and pain. They are effective for mild to moderate pain, but can irritate the stomach lining, cause nausea, and in rare cases cause kidney damage. They can also stir up trouble with gastritis and ulcers.

Painkillers

Narcotics are powerful painkillers and may be prescribed for pain relief. Science has searched for pain relief for many centuries. Opium is one of the oldest painkillers known to humankind. In the 1800s morphine, named after Morpheus, the Greek god of dreams, was first purified from opium. It decreased opium's nasty side effects and increased its painkilling properties. In the beginning, morphine was used as an anesthesia prior to operations. Patients needed to be anesthetized with rather large doses, which led to other problems. (As you know, both opium and morphine are highly addictive.)

Man still continues the quest for the perfect drug, yet some ancient truths still apply: Painkillers may mask the pain and give temporary relief, but *they do not alleviate the problem*. If you take painkillers for any amount of time, possible abuse of the drug and addiction need to be monitored, preferably by yourself, and if not, by your doctor.

As the user's tolerance to a narcotic increases, the doses need to be increased to obtain the same effect. Drugs that fall into this category include codeine, morphine, Darvon, and Demerol.

Your doctor may prescribe acetaminophen (Tylenol) for pain. Tylenol is a moderate painkiller that may, if taken in large quantities, upset your stomach, but it is not addictive.

Side effects of narcotics include addiction, sedation, and loss of sex drive if taken long term.

Muscle Relaxants

Many physicians avoid muscle relaxants. Muscle relaxants work on much the same principle as painkillers. Sometimes the two are prescribed simultaneously. Parafon, Flexeril, and Valium are commonly prescribed muscle relaxants. Muscle relaxants do exactly what they say: They relax you. The extended use of these powerful relaxants can produce depression, and one of the side effects is drowsiness. Muscle relaxants are addictive if abused.

Drugs for Depression

Depression understandably may be wedded to long-term pain and is often associated with sleeping difficulties. Serotonin, a chemical produced in the brain, is also associated with depression, chronic pain, and sleep disturbances. Certain antidepressants are used to help serotonin levels in the brain return to normal. Antidepressants take a few weeks to begin working. They don't activate overnight.

Newer antidepressants on the market are not habit forming. Side effects may include weight gain, grogginess, dry mouth, and in some cases, constipation.

Referencing Drugs

How many times have you taken a drug like tetracycline, gone and soaked up a few rays, and come home with spots all over your body? A reaction to the drug? Not really. Tetracycline is photosensitive and does not mix well with sunshine. Nevertheless, this frightening side effect is often not noted by the hurried physician or busy pharmacist. Of course, the small print on the prescription advises you not to go in the sun. But did you read it?

So what's the point? When taking drugs for pain, know their potency, side effects, and what they mix and don't mix with. Frankly, your doctor probably doesn't have the time, or may not even know everything there is to know about the drug. But there are drug references to help you, and you'll find them in libraries as well as pharmacies. The following are excellent guides to help you understand the drug or drugs you are taking.

The Physician's Desk Reference, which provides detailed labeling information but may not give other information easily understood.

The Complete Drug Reference, published by Consumer Reports Books.

The Essential Guide to Prescription Drugs, by James W. Long, M.D., and James J. Rybacki, Pharm.D., published by Harper Perennial; an excellent source.

A Complete Guide to Prescription & Non-Prescription Drugs, by H. Winter Griffith, M.D., published by The Body Press/Perigee; pictorials make it easy to quickly access information.

What You Need to Know

When referencing a drug, ask the following:

- Is the drug generic? If so, this certainly will give you some pricing options.

- What class of drug is it: mild analgesic, tranquilizer, anti-inflammatory?

- What different brand names categorize this drug?

- What are the principal uses of the drug? To relieve pain for musculoskeletal problems? For acute pain? Osteoarthritis? Fever reduction?

- Do you take the drug on an empty stomach, or with food, or water, or must you remain upright for thirty minutes after taking it?

- Do you have an ulcer or asthma, or a blood-cell disorder? Some drugs cannot be taken with existing conditions.

- What are the side effects? Will you become drowsy, irritable, or nauseated?

- Precautions. Does the drug affect pregnant or breast-feeding women, or elderly adults?
- Is the drug habit-forming?

Ultimately, if you are taking several drugs for different purposes, keep a chart of the drugs, and how they affect you. Store drugs separately. Your doctor may prescribe the drugs, but you are the guardian of what you pop in your mouth; this is *your* responsibility.

To better understand the expertise that each specialist brings to the back field, turn the page. You might control your own back pain and never set foot in a specialist's office, but if you have a herniated disk, degenerative spine disease, or an injury, chances are you'll see more than one back expert in your quest to understand what happened and how to rectify it.

Chapter 7

THE SPECIALIST

Ferreting out the perfect solution for your back problem requires time. Despite the prevalence of the problem, there appears to be no consensus among clinicians on how to treat it. Sometimes you find the right clinician to treat your back problem, and the result is instant success. But the more common scenario is that you do not strike it lucky on the first round. If this is the case, running the gamut of back doctors can be frustrating and isolating.

Today, a variety of doctors, philosophies, education, and treatment await the back-pain sufferer. Each specialist provides a particular level of expertise. Unless you are badly injured or suffer from a fracture or break, however, chances are you will commence at the primary level of practitioners.

GENERAL PRACTITIONER OR INTERNIST

Since back pain is such a common malady, one might assume that your general practitioner or internist is an expert when it comes to treating your back. This isn't necessarily true. Nevertheless, starting with your primary physician is the place to rule out other problems that may affect your spine, such as referred pain, or pain originating elsewhere in your body that may afflict the back. Certainly, if you belong to an HMO or are a first-time back statistic, you will most likely be referred to your general practitioner or internist. He or she will take a complete medical history and run tests to rule out infections that may concurrently occur. A course of pain medication, rest, and exercise will probably be advised. While a general practitioner or internist is not a back specialist, he or she can diagnose a pinched nerve or disease that may produce back pain. Many times, a trip to your primary caregiver resolves the problem. But if it doesn't, you will be referred to a specialist.

OSTEOPATHS

Osteopaths surfaced around the time of chiropractics, although statistically there is only one practicing osteopath for every three chiropractors in the United States. Osteopaths practice medicine differently today than they did a hundred years ago. Traditionally trained to look at how the internal organs such as the heart or liver interact with the musculoskeletal system, osteopaths had and still have extraordinary palpitatory skills. With the advent of diagnostic tests, today's back problems are less likely to be diagnosed by skilled hands.

All osteopaths are trained as general practitioners and are well-rounded physicians in the sense that their training looks at the whole individual rather than one special area. Ideally, they can diagnose many different conditions and treat them effectively. An osteopath looks at a patient's environment, such as stress or accidents, along with the psychosocial as well as the physical factors. While osteopaths are skilled practitioners in manual treatment and take a therapeutic approach to the practice of medicine, including all forms of medical therapy and diagnoses, like all doctors, they have individual approaches. Even though an osteopath may prescribe drugs or surgery, his or her emphasis is on the relationship of the organs and the musculoskeletal system. They recognize and correct structural problems using different types of manipulation. An osteopath takes a more holistic approach to medicine than a surgeon, internist, or orthopedist and emphasizes the curative benefits of spinal manipulation.

If you recall Audrey's experience with her ruptured disk in chapter 2, it was the osteopath who finally relieved her pain. Until she ruptured her disk, she knew nothing about osteopathic medicine. Today she highly regards the osteopath as the savior of her back.

PHYSICAL THERAPIST

A physical therapist is not a doctor but holds a degree in physical therapy. A physical therapist follows a program recommended by a medical doctor. Legally, physical therapists must have a prescribed treatment by a physician before treating a patient. Physical therapists work manually on soft tissue, joints, and muscles. They teach body mechanics and are often the educator when it comes to your back. Good physical therapists teach you how to move through daily activities with a bum back. They evaluate your posture, sitting, job tasks, and body mechanics, and instruct you on how to protect your back. They teach stretching and mobilization, and ideally work with you on an individual basis. They may administer heat, ice, or ultrasound and are guardians of your rehabilitation progress. Physical therapists chart your progress and help you to alter aspects of your life that are hard on your back.

Today many physical therapists specialize only in spine and neck care. If physical therapy is part of your back program, seek a physical therapist who specializes in the spine, not someone who has taken a quick weekend course and claims spine specialization. It is best to ask what credentials your physical therapist has, and for how long, when it comes to spine care. Ideally, a physical therapist should be affiliated with a spine-care center.

Depending on the severity of your problem, even the best of general practitioners, osteopaths, and physical therapists may not be able to solve what ails your back. If you are not one of the 90 percent who recover from your back trauma in six weeks, you may seek another level of expertise—your secondary caregivers.

PHYSIATRIST

You may never hear the word *physiatrist* until you injure your back or have a stroke. A physiatrist is an M.D. who specializes in musculoskeletal rehabilitation, stroke management, and spinal cord injuries. Some physiatrists have a subspecialty in sports medicine. Some can administer injections, such as an epidural, or prescribe braces. Physiatrists are adept at rehabilitating a variety of medical problems, including injuries, postoperative difficulties, and movement dysfunction. Experts in nonoperative treatment, physiatrists adhere to an exercise program for your back. State-of-the-art spine-care centers all have physiatrists on board.

ORTHOPEDIST OR ORTHOPEDIC SURGEON

An orthopedist is an M.D. or D.O. whose specialties are bone, joints, and muscle disorders. They often see patients at all three levels of care: primary, secondary, and tertiary. They treat a range of maladies, from the straightforward, first-time herniated disk with a pinched nerve to intense spine abnormality and traumatic injuries to psychological adjustments related to spine disorders. Orthopedists may prescribe drugs or request a complete workup to include a standard orthopedic neurological test, a CAT scan, or an MRI. If you need surgery of any kind, or have spinal stenosis or a ruptured disk, it is the orthopedic surgeon you will see. While many equate orthopedic surgeons with going under the knife, orthopedic surgeons often treat back pain nonsurgically and conservatively.

NEUROLOGIST AND NEUROSURGEON

A neurologist is an M.D. with a specialty in treating neurological disorders nonsurgically. Neurologists diagnose and treat disorders of the brain, spine, nerve tissue, and peripheral nerves. A neurosurgeon is a specialist in the same disorders, but is also licensed to practice neurological surgery. Up until the last two decades, neurosurgeons dominated spine surgery. The orthopedist treated patients but didn't operate on their spines. Today, orthopedists who specialize in spine care dominate surgery and conservative spine care.

PSYCHIATRIST

A psychiatrist is a doctor of psychiatry, not to be confused with a psychologist, who is not an M.D. A good spine-care center will have a psychiatrist on staff, and many centers also house a psychologist. Why would anyone need a psychiatrist for a ruptured disk? Most likely, you won't need a psychiatrist for a ruptured disk. But if you suffer chronic pain in your spine or must manage intense pain and disability related to an injury, a psychiatrist may be very helpful. When an individual suffers from chronic back pain, the entire family suffers. Often, the person dealing with pain cannot manage to translate to those closest to him or her what is occurring psychologically or physically. The psychiatrist or sometimes the psychologist works with either the individual patient or the family. A psychiatrist, being an M.D., may prescribe drugs, while a psychologist may not.

Whether your back problem demands a single visit to your general practitioner or requires the expertise of an osteopath or an orthopedic surgeon, diagnostic tests will be used to both pinpoint and clinically further the understanding of the problem plaguing your spine. Chapter 8 offers an overview of current diagnostic testing procedures and how they differ.

Chapter 8

TYPES OF STANDARDIZED TESTS

What may be standard treatment for one back may not be standard for another. While there are several tests for back problems, it's wise to ask yourself and your practitioner a few questions before embarking on a series of diagnostic procedures. Foremost, do you absolutely require the procedure? Are there risks involved? Is the procedure painful, and are there side effects? Did you know that except for life-threatening emergencies, you are the person to authorize tests, not your doctor? Many individuals fail to inquire about a test; they simply accept that the doctor has ordered it. Doctors are aware that they have a legal obligation to explain potential hazards or risks, but if they aren't forthcoming with information, it's up to you to ask. Many times you must sign a release before a test is administered. Read the fine print. If you have reservations about any test, discuss it with your doctor before proceeding. A second opinion is always a good idea if you are having misgivings about the type of test recommended. The following procedures are often part of the diagnostic window to help doctors clearly understand your back problem. Some procedures are more frequently used than others.

X RAY

The X ray still remains a standard test with most practitioners. Why do doctors bother with X rays while there are so many more sophisticated high-tech choices for detecting spinal disorders? Primarily, X rays are relatively low in cost and are a prudent choice both physically and medically. Spine X rays are commonly used to evaluate neck and back injuries or persistent numbness. An X ray shows only bone, not soft tissue. And as you well understand, if bone is not the significant culprit causing problems in your spine—and the majority of the time it is not—nothing will show up on film. This is the greatest limitation with this type of test. On the brighter side, an X ray can rule out other possibilities, such as tumors or referred complications. In a major departure from traditional practice, federal health officials convened by the Agency for Health Care Policy and Research recently released a study suggesting that expensive tests used to diagnose low back pain may be useless unless symptoms indicate fractures, tumors, infections, or spinal nerve-root problems. While not everyone may agree with the findings, unless your practitioner suspects an urgent spinal complication, he or she will start with an X ray. The procedure takes about twenty minutes and requires removal of all jewelry. The greatest concern with X rays is exposure to radiation. If you're pregnant, carefully weigh the risk factor. If your back trouble disappears within a few weeks, you won't need other tests. On the other hand, if the pain intensifies and your condition worsens, the X ray is just the beginning in your search.

CAT SCAN

A computed axial tomography reveals high-quality cross-sectional images of the spine or area in question. You lie on a table while the technician, who remains behind a glass, uses a computer-guided X-ray tube. Although you must sit still, the procedure is painless. You can hear the rotation or clicking of the scanner as the machine rotates. Sometimes the technician will help you change positions to obtain a better image. The drawback with this type of test is that you are exposed to radiation. Inform your doctor if you have a reaction to shellfish; sometimes a dye is used in the scan that such people cannot tolerate. Obviously, if you are pregnant, you may want to consider skipping this diagnostic test, or else discuss alternatives with your doctor. The CAT scan remains a good tool for evaluating herniated disks, spinal stenosis, or injuries to the bones. Tumors, degenerative bone diseases, and spinal infections are visible in a CAT scan.

Compared with the X ray, CAT scans are costly, but they are a much better tool for evaluating more invasive problems related to the spine.

MRI

Magnetic resonance imaging, a noninvasive test conducted without radiation, is considered a gold mine in high-quality testing. The patient must lie quietly in a large, body-length tube while being scanned. The procedure can run from an hour and a half to two hours. It's painless. The scan visualizes tissue with a magnetic field recording that uses high-speed computers to provide very clear images of the spine and other tissue. The MRI is effective for visualizing soft-tissue disorders, disk disease, tumors, infections, and spinal nerve compression from stenosis and nerve disorders. The MRI can see through bone. It uses a powerful magnetic field and radio-frequency energy to produce images. The images are monitored by a computer, which processes the images on a video screen for interpretation. While your entire body lies perfectly still in the tube, the scan examines only the area of your spine in question. It does not scan the entire body. The room is very quiet, and you can hear the sounds of the scanner machine. The technician produces the images with special equipment. You have no direct contact with the equipment. There are no known harmful effects with an MRI.

Claustrophobia may be a concern, since you are cooped up inside that tube. The MRI cannot be conducted on women with intrauterine devices (IUDs) or individuals with metal implants or pacemakers. The estimated cost for an MRI is considerable: around $1,000.

EMG

An electromyogram is an invasive test administered by a specialist. The test measures the speed of motor-nerve conduction. Fine wires or electrodes are inserted into muscles and nerves and then electrically stimulated. The purpose of the test is to help diagnose nerve disorders and to differentiate between primary muscle disorders. This technique determines which nerve is injured and if the injury occurred recently. You will be asked not to smoke for twenty-four hours prior to the test and to refrain from caffeine intake for several hours before. Inform your doctor if you are taking medications.

An electromyograph machine detects and measures response. A needle is inserted into the selected area. A sharp, brief pain ensues each time the needle electrode is reinserted. The muscle or nerve's electrical potential is measured during rest and contraction and is displayed on a screen. The procedure may be a bit uncomfortable and lasts approximately one hour.

Blocks

Blocks, an injection of corticosteroids administered into the site of pain are useful when the amount of pain is severe. They can be used in diagnostic treatment of chronic problems, but tend to be more effective with such acute problems as pinched nerves.

The steroid in the block reduces inflammation, which is critical. If, for example, a pinched nerve is not remedied, blood supply is cut off, resulting in permanent tissue damage. The injection cuts the swelling so that the blood supply can flow normally. A block will not change the structure of the problem, such as a pinched nerve, but it will buy time, allowing the body to heal. If successful—and statistically between 70 and 85 percent are—the block allows for a modicum of normality while the body heals. If the block is not successful, the individual must repose until the inflammation diminishes and further tests are taken.

Blocks have been widely used for the last decade. While there are subcategories to blocks, the two types commonly used today are epidural and facet blocks. Facet blocks are injected into the facet. Epidural blocks are injected into epidural space. An anesthesiologist, surgeon, or physiatrist can perform these procedures.

The procedures consist of injecting corticosteroids with a solution into the spine. Alternately, the steroid may be taken orally. The steroid remains in your body for approximately six weeks. Some individuals report very little pain, others insist the procedure is painful. For the person dealing with long-term pain, there may already be a nerve sensitivity in the area, thus creating an uncomfortable experience. If the individual responds well to the injection, relief comes within seventy-two hours. If not, a second or third injection from a different approach may be more successful. Sometimes there is no response. Some physicians administer blocks in a series of three injections.

But since the solution remains in your body for six weeks, this may not be necessary. The only rationale for a second block is if the first one doesn't work. So consider this if a second or third injection is offered.

Blocks are sometimes performed to pinpoint pain or to glean information about the area in question. Although a local anesthetic is given, the individual must remain awake to communicate his or her response to the needle. The needle must be moved, and, because anything in this region is hypersensitive, this can hurt.

In general, blocks are not a risky procedure. As in any invasive procedure, protecting the nerves is always the main concern. Blocks may or may not be done with X rays or a fluoroscope machine. They are always performed in a clinic or hospital. Costs run between $250 and $800, depending on where the block is performed, and who is administering it.

MYELOGRAM

This invasive procedure examines the fluid-filled sac that lies around the nerves and spinal cord in your spinal canal. The myelogram at one time was used in locating and identifying such problems as a herniated intervertebral disk, tumors, or injuries to the nerve roots branching off the spinal cord. Today, an MRI scan is performed either in place of or prior to a myelogram, since the myelogram is an invasive procedure and carries a slight risk of adverse reaction. An MRI may be a more prudent procedure, although in some cases a myelogram and CAT scan give the most information.

Instruction to avoid food but to take plenty of liquids is given prior to the test. You may be given a sedative or injection to relax. You lie facedown, and the site of the procedure is anesthetized with a local anesthetic. A longer needle then protrudes into the spinal canal and a small amount of fluid is taken from the spine and sent to the lab for analysis. The position of the needle is monitored by a fluoroscope, which is connected to a screen. A contrasting X-ray dye is injected into fluid-filled space that surrounds the spinal cord. You are tilted under a fluoroscope so that the dye can be observed. X rays follow. The body absorbs the water-based dye.

You must sit up or lie with your head elevated for six to eight hours after the procedure. Although you'll leave the hospital or clinic the same day, plan to rest a few days after this procedure. Some complain that this is a painful experience, while others report a headache afterward, or some discomfort as the needle goes in. Side effects include nausea, headaches, vomiting, and post-procedure infection at the injection site. Myelograms may be followed by a CAT scan while the dye is still present to pinpoint the exact location and degree of herniation.

DISCOGRAM

A discogram is a surgical staging test to try and identify which disk or disks are problematic or abnormal. It is frequently painful, and spine surgeons or anesthesiologists and radiologists perform it. There is a risk of disk infection in one in five hundred procedures.

BONE SCAN

A bone scan is a procedure in which an injection of radioactive material travels through the bloodstream to attach itself to the bone. This material moves to areas that are either actively breaking down bone or are making new bone. It shows up in large amounts in areas of abnormal bone and detects the early signs of bone cancer, infection, or fractures. The bone scan helps evaluate unexplained bone pain or abnormalities found on regular X rays. The test is done in the department of nuclear medicine, and although it does not require an overnight stay, it is lengthy. After the radioactive substance is injected into your veins, you must wait approximately three hours for the material to distribute throughout your body. Drinking a massive amount of water is required to clear the body of radioactive material not involved with the bone tissue. The actual scan takes about one hour, as you lie on your back and the camera moves slowly back and forth above your body. Infants, pregnant women, and breast-feeding mothers are not good candidates for this procedure. A bone scan is expensive and is not done routinely.

You may never have cause for more than an X ray or an MRI. If, however, tumors or certain infections invade your body, several of these tests may be helpful. Chapter 9 discusses infections and rare tumors that may invade the spinal area.

Chapter 9

INFECTIONS AND TUMORS

There are a few rare infections and even rarer cancers that affect the back. This chapter discusses the types of infections that can occur in the spine and cancers that may be associated with the spine. Then why, you ask, even discuss the doom and gloom of infections and tumors in a sourcebook on back pain, if they so rarely occur? The reality is they do occur, and while they may be atypical for the majority of the population experiencing back ailments, infections and tumors are serious, and once diagnosed must be treated accordingly. Second, any infection or tumor located in the spinal area is like a thorn. If unattended, it slowly, or sometimes quickly, impinges its will elsewhere in the body.

Osteomyelitis can occur if bacteria in the bloodstream reach the vertebral bodies. Vertebral osteomyelitis occurs infrequently in healthy adults. Certain conditions appear to predispose one to vertebral osteomyelitis, the most common of which is diabetes. With diabetes, the weakened immune response makes one more prone to infection. Intravenous drug users also have an increased vulnerability to this infection.

Many cases of vertebral osteomyelitis result from another or related source of infection, and are spread by circulation of the bloodstream. Commonly, the primary infection sites are the genitourinary tract or pelvic organs. The staphylococcus aureus organism is usually the infectious culprit. Peak ages for this infection are during childhood and in adulthood between ages fifty and sixty.

Symptoms of vertebral osteomyelitis are low-grade to very severe prolonged back pain. Chronic osteomyelitis, if left untreated, causes acute attacks of pain and fever. Antibiotics are the primary form of treatment in the early stages; if left untreated, however, surgery may be indicated.

TUBERCULOSIS

Tuberculosis, once considered an erradicated infectious disease, is back. Tuberculosis, an acute or chronic bacterial infection most frequently found in the lungs, is caused by either *Mycobacterium tuberculosis* or *Mycobacterium bovis*, bacteria passed to humans through dairy products. Like a cold, the infection is spread through airborne droplets breathed out into the air by an infected person. In the lungs, the bacteria form masses of tissue called tubercles. Coughing, breathing impairment, and sputum are early symptoms. Since 1984, tuberculosis has been on the rise, especially among the elderly and in children. Tuberculosis may recur after a latent period if not treated properly. And while it is most common in the lungs, TB also exists in the kidneys, bones, spinal area, lymph nodes, and membranes surrounding the brain. In rare cases, it can spread throughout the entire body and can cause a spinal infection if the organism that carries the disease reaches the vertebral bodies. Tuberculosis of the spine, called Pott's disease, begins gradually and involves weight loss and pain in the spinal nerve root. If not treated, it may result in paralysis.

While tuberculosis has been a disease common to underdeveloped countries, it's on the rise in the United States. The Centers for Disease Control in Atlanta, Georgia, currently estimates that a million people worldwide have been infected with tuberculosis. A standard skin test is required of all school-age children, pregnant women, and individuals working in restaurant and health-care professions in this country. If a tuberculin test is positive and the individual has tuberculosis, the condition is treated with antibiotic therapy for approximately two weeks. Hospitalization is not usually necessary.

MENINGITIS

The doctor said her son had the flu. Linnea spent the weekend by her twenty-one-month-old's bedside. But David didn't respond to anything; he seemed listless. Monday, Linnea returned to the pediatrician. One look at David's stiff body, particularly the neck, confirmed the doctor's suspicion. He told Linnea to bundle up David, and the three of them drove to the hospital. A spinal tap confirmed David had meningitis. The pediatrician spent several hours explaining the potentially dangerous side effects. David spent two weeks in the hospital on intravenous antibiotic. Linnea still recalls the nightmare.

"David was crabby, cried constantly, and flinched at the slightest touch when we changed his diaper. His muscle coordination was obviously impaired, and his back and hips hurt, but the worst news was yet to come."

David's father, Ken, was the first to suspect his son was not responding to his voice when he tried feeding him. The nurses assured Ken that David was fine, just in a lot of pain. But a brain-stem test confirmed Ken's fear. David had lost his hearing.

Today David communicates through sign language and works with a speech therapist. After years of physical therapy, David's motor skills have improved immensely. He rides his bike to school, swims, and is a member of the Boy Scouts. He's like many normal ten-year-old boys.

What Is Meningitis?

Meningitis is an inflammation of the tissues that cover the brain and spinal cord. It's rare, but it's very serious. Highly contagious, it seems to occur mainly in children under the age of five, or older adults. The most serious kind of meningitis is caused by bacteria. Several different types of bacteria are involved. Children under the age of two are at greatest risk for this form of meningitis. Meningitis can also be caused by viruses and other organisms, such as fungi or parasites. The viral form is not as serious.

The bacteria are often found in the mouths and throats of healthy children. This does not mean these children will get meningitis; that occurs only when the bacteria reach the bloodstream.

Before antibiotics, 90 percent of the children with meningitis died. The 10 percent who survived had retardation, deafness, or convulsions. Today the outlook is brighter.

With prompt diagnosis, 70 percent of those who get meningitis recover without complications. Even serious cases have only minor complications, with hearing loss the most prevalent. Meningitis must be detected early and treated aggressively with massive doses of antibiotics in order to be cured. If meningitis is even suspected, doctors often start a patient on antibiotics as a prophylactic measure.

Symptoms

In a child less than two months old, the presence of fever, decreased appetite, listlessness, or increased crying warrant a call to your doctor. Meningitis can be very subtle at this age. From two months to two years, which is the most common age for meningitis, symptoms are fever, nausea, vomiting, decreased appetite, excessive crankiness, or excessive drowsiness. Older children will have the above symptoms but may also complain of headache, pain in the back, or a stiff neck.

If your pediatrician suspects meningitis, he or she will perform a blood test and obtain some spinal fluid via a spine tap.

Today, some types of bacterial meningitis can be prevented with vaccines or antibiotics. In David's case, ten years ago, pediatricians didn't have an inoculation against meningitis until a child reached the age of two. Now, a new vaccine allows pediatricians to inoculate in the first year of life. This is probably the best prevention against meningitis, although it is not 100 percent effective.

HERPES ZOSTER OR SHINGLES

Jean, a spry, active woman, was seventy-eight years old when her sight failed. So disconcerted over the impinging loss, she didn't pay attention to the pain in her shoulder. But in a matter of a few weeks, her shoulder began to itch and constantly pulsate with pain. Her doctor couldn't find anything wrong. It was Jean's optometrist who diagnosed shingles. The diagnosis was the beginning of a painful nightmare. Jean spent three months sleeping in the big chair in her living room. She couldn't lie down.

"I had shingles running down the back of my head, shoulders, and all over my back. I couldn't sleep, never mind lie down. Agonizing pain made the simplest activity impossible. I've never experienced such hell. I've had two colostomies, and the pain with those was a picnic compared with the shingles."

Jean's shingles lasted three months. Painkillers didn't work, although several of her friends suffering from shingles had prescriptions for medications that seemed to ease their pain.

"I waited it out," recalls Jean. "I switched doctors, but oddly enough, neither my doctor nor optometrist suggested shingles had anything to do with losing my eyesight. My sight is gone, and I have residual marks from the shingles, but thankfully, I've not had another episode of shingles. I don't think I could live through it."

What Are Shingles?

Herpes zoster is a common cause of back pain in the elderly and individuals with weakened immune systems. Herpes zoster, commonly called shingles, is caused by the same virus responsible for chicken pox: varicella. It is a cousin of the viruses that cause genital herpes and cold sores. It is not the virus that causes AIDS. When people contract chicken pox, the virus is disseminated throughout the body. During the acute phase of the illness, most of the viral organisms are destroyed, but a few hide in the sensory nerves. In approximately 10 to 20 percent of those who have had chicken pox around the fifth decade of life, as one's immune system weakens, the virus can resurface with a painful vengeance.

Musculoskeletal pain can precede the more common skin symptoms of a red rash, characterized by small, fluid-filled blisters, by weeks or months. Often shingles goes undiagnosed if there is no rash with the back pain. The virus is painful, described as an intense burning, itching, or stabbing sensation. Fatigue and low-grade fever can accompany the pain. Once the blisters emerge, they last for approximately two to three weeks. When the rash disappears and the blisters heal, the virus is no longer active. About 20 percent of those suffering with shingles and who are over age sixty have some nerve damage creating chronic pain near the site of the rash. This pain, known as postherpetic neuralgia, is a condition that can go on for years.

The virus is contagious through direct contact during the blister stage and can cause chicken pox in people who aren't already immune. In a few people, the virus attacks the eyes, and in immune-compromised individuals, the virus can invade the lungs or brain. Unlike a cold, you cannot catch shingles directly by sitting next to someone who has shingles.

What can you do for shingles? In the early stages, an analgesic such as aspirin may help. More severe pain may require painkillers. High doses of acyclovir, a prescription medication for shingles, may reduce the rash. The drawback is that the drug is expensive and must be taken forty-eight hours after the rash first appears. Over-the-counter topical cream, Capsaicin, derived from red pepper, helps some with pain relief. It is also expensive, about $70 for a one-month supply. Some individuals report temporary relief with transcutaneous electrical nerve stimulation (TENS), electrical pulses that beam through the skin via a portable instrument. Other drugs on the market, such as antidepressants and anticonvulsants, are sometimes prescribed for chronic shingles. In extremely painful cases, some individuals opt for a nerve block, a local anesthetic injected into or around the infected nerve. This numbs the area for several hours, bringing temporary relief.

Recently the FDA approved a chicken pox vaccine for infants that stimulates an immune response. Many doctors have started inoculating infants with the vaccine. Nevertheless, in some circles the question still remains: Will the weakened vaccine itself, once injected into the body, actually provoke shingles in the future?

TUMORS AND CANCER

Every knowledgeable doctor will tell you this: Cancer of the spine is rare. Cancer rarely starts in the spine, but can spread to the spine from its primary site via the spine's extensive blood supply. By the time a cancer reaches the spine, it is already present somewhere else in your body. Since the inception of this book, by sheer coincidence I have had occasion to know two people who were diagnosed with cancer in their spines, and who subsequently died. The two individuals had opposite lifestyles and types of cancer, and they battled and treated their cancers differently. Both went to their doctor because of unrelenting pain in their backs, but neither of the individual's cancer originated in the spine. While this chapter discusses the most prevalent types of cancers and tumors that may be affiliated with the spine, do keep in mind that they are extremely rare. Less than 1 percent of those seeking a doctor for back problems have a tumor or cancer. If your back is bothering you for an extended period of time, get it checked to rule out the worst.

What Are Tumors?

Tumors are abnormal cell growth. Cells normally divide and replace themselves in an orderly, controlled fashion. When cell division becomes disorderly or out of control, too many cells are produced. Abnormal growth occurs, forming a mass of tissue known as a tumor.

There are two types of tumors: benign (noncancerous) and malignant (cancerous). Benign tumors are more common than malignant ones. Benign tumors limit their growth to one area; malignant tumors do not, and they metastasize elsewhere.

The following types of cancer may present themselves in the back or spinal area. They may also show up elsewhere in your body without afflicting the spine.

Multiple Myeloma

According to the National Cancer Institute, 12,000 Americans are diagnosed with multiple myeloma. Multiple myeloma is a type of cancer that affects certain white blood cells called plasma cells. Plasma cells are part of the immune system. All white blood cells begin their development in the bone marrow, which is a spongy tissue in the center of the bone. These cells produce antibodies. When types of cancer involve the plasma cells, the body keeps producing more and more cells. The unneeded abnormal cells are called myeloma cells. These cells tend to collect in the bone marrow. In some instances, the cells collect in only one bone, forming a single mass, or plasmacytoma. Usually, though, the myeloma cells collect in many bones, creating the condition called multiple myeloma.

As myeloma cells increase, they damage and weaken bone, causing fractures. Damaged bones release calcium into the blood, creating a condition called hypercalcemia, causing loss of appetite, nausea, muscle weakness, and restlessness. Because the bone marrow cannot form normal plasma cells, infection sets in. Due to excess antibody proteins and calcium, an individual with myeloma may have kidney complications.

Symptoms of multiple myeloma vary depending on how advanced the disease is. When symptoms occur, the pain may arise in the bones, often in the back or ribs. Broken bones, weight loss, or fatigue may also occur. In the advanced stage, symptoms are vomiting, problems with urination, and numbness in the legs. The urination problems and leg numbness may have nothing to do with cancer but be the result of the back problems.

If an individual has bone pain, X rays may show fractures. A bone scan, MRI, or bone marrow aspiration may follow. Treatment depends on the extent of cancer in the body and can be complex. Oncologists, hematologists, and radiation oncologists are all doctors who specialize in this disease.

Multiple myeloma is not easy to cure; chemotherapy is traditionally the treatment of choice. Many individuals take chemotherapy, or systemic therapy, by mouth or injections. The drugs are given in cycles, followed by a rest period. Most individuals take chemotherapy at home or in the doctor's office. Side effects include lower resistance to infection, loss of appetite, hair loss, and vomiting. Fatigue, swelling, and indigestion may also be involved. These side effects usually disappear when treatment is finished. Sometimes a person with a tumor made up of cancerous plasma cells, the aforementioned plasmacytoma, receives local therapy or radiation.

With radiation, high-energy rays are aimed at the tumor, affecting local cells in the area. Sometimes individuals with multiple myeloma receive both forms of treatment. Radiation causes a person to be more tired than usual. Radiation in the lower back may cause nausea, vomiting, or diarrhea, due to the lower digestive tract being exposed to radiation. Side effects usually disappear after therapy is over.

Bone Cancers

Cancer that begins in the bone is called primary bone cancer and is quite rare. Pain is the most frequent symptom of this type of cancer, which usually presents itself in the arms and legs but may be present elsewhere. Children and young adults are more likely to have bone cancer than adults. Again, cancers of the bone are rare, with only about 2,000 new cases diagnosed in the United States each year, according to the National Cancer Institute. This translates to one case in 100,000 people. Scientists do not know what causes bone cancer.

Osteosarcoma is most commonly diagnosed between the ages of ten and twenty-five. It affects males more than females and occurs in the ends of the bones, during the peak years of bone growth. In adults, it often strikes people who have a history of Paget's disease, a noncancerous condition characterized by abnormal development of new bone cells. There is some speculation that osteosarcoma might be triggered by overactivity of bone cells. Research does indicate that children who have been treated with radiation or anticancer drugs for other types of cancer are at risk for bone tumors.

Pain is the first symptom of bone cancer. Tumors near the joints cause stiffness. Tumors near the spine can affect bladder or bowel function. Your doctor will check the tissue attached to the bone and order a blood test to determine if there is an overabundance of alkaline phosphatase, an enzyme produced by cells that form new bone tissue. Various types of diagnostic tests may follow, such as bone scans or CAT scans. A surgical biopsy concludes whether a bone tumor is malignant or benign.

Surgery is the primary form of treatment for most bone cancers, to remove the primary tumor and surrounding tissue. Amputation, once considered the most effective treatment, is being replaced by preoperative and postoperative chemotherapy. Chemotherapy is used for nonmetastatic osteosarcoma to destroy cancer cells that may have blocked the bloodstream.

Ewing's sarcoma, usually present in people between ten and twenty-five years of age, most often affects teenagers. Forming in the middle of the bone, this cancer affects long bones and can occur in the ribs. Ewing's sarcoma develops primarily in bone marrow. While it causes less destruction of the bone, its entrance into the bloodstream allows it to travel to other parts of the body quickly. Because of the tendency for Ewing's sarcoma to metastasize quickly, surgery is usually not successful. Ewing's sarcoma responds best to chemotherapy and radiation treatment.

Chondro sarcoma, confined to adults, is a condition in which tumors form around the cartilage and rubbery joint tissue. It occurs less frequently than osteosarcoma, but more frequently than Ewing's sarcoma. It is treated in much the same way as osteosarcoma. Once again, these cancers occur infrequently.

Spinal Cord Tumors

Spinal cord tumors are not common, although 10,000 Americans develop primary or metastatic spinal cord tumors each year. The spinal cord is like a living cable. It contains bundles of nerves that relay messages from the brain to nerves throughout the body. A tumor near the spinal cord can inhibit this communication. A tumor exerting pressure on the spinal cord or the nerves restricts the cord's supply of blood. This in turn causes pain, sensory change, and motor problems. The parts of the body affected by these symptoms depend upon where in the spinal cord the tumor is located.

Symptoms may be constant severe pain, with a burning, aching sensation. Loss of sensation or numbness may also occur. Because nerves control muscles, a number of muscle-related problems may arise, such as stiffness, spasticity, or bladder impairment. Generally, symptoms occur near the area of the tumor. If you have a tumor in the thoracic spine, for example, pain may be felt in the chest, intensifying when you sneeze or cough. A tumor in the lower spine can cause back or leg pain. In most parts of the body, benign tumors are not particularly harmful. This isn't always the case in the spinal cord, which is the central nervous system's primary partner.

Spinal tumors are divided into three groups: *extradural* tumors that occur between the bony spinal canal and the dura mater, which protects the spinal cord; *intradural* tumors, which grow inside the dura; and those that grow outside the spinal cord, called *extramedullary* tumors, or *intramedullary* tumors that grow inside the spinal cord.

If a spinal tumor is suspected, your doctor will conduct a neurological exam to check reflexes, hearing, sensation, balance, and coordination. A CAT scan, MRI, or PET (positron emission tomography, which provides a picture of brain activity) may be taken. A spinal tap will also be conducted.

Three common treatments for spinal cord tumors include surgery, radiation, and chemotherapy. If the tumor is operable, or placed where it will not cause neurological damage, several types of surgeries are applicable, depending on the tumor.

With microsurgery, surgeons use a high-powered microscope to magnify the view of the area being operated on. Stereotactic procedures use computers to create a three-dimensional map to help surgeons approach difficult areas with greater precision. Lasers can destroy tissue by beaming concentrated light energy to destroy it, while ultrasonic aspirators use sound waves to break up tumors, then aspirate them.

Radiation therapy bombards the tumor to destroy the tumorous cells. Chemotherapy involves drugs that are taken orally or injected into the bloodstream in order to kill cells that are growing and dividing.

Because spinal cord tumors are difficult to diagnose, and because they occur in the most sensitive area in your body, their treatment demands great skill and expertise. Choosing a highly trained physician familiar with spinal cord tumors may be one of the most important decisions you ever make. Refer to the appendix for more information regarding tumors and infections.

Meningoioms

Meningoioms, or benign tumors, are twice as common in women as in men. They occur in the thoracic spine on one side of the spinal column and may cause back pain.

While the majority of you will never have to consider treatment for tumors or make decisions about surgery for tumors, according to statistics, a number of you have or will experience back surgery in your lifetime. Why do so many Americans undergo back surgery once, twice, or half a dozen times? Why doesn't back surgery always relieve a herniated disk, or sciatica? If these questions are of any concern, or if you are contemplating back surgery or a second surgery, turn the page.

Chapter 10

SPINE SURGERY

Judith remembers precisely the moment that left her incapacitated for two and a half years. She moved a dresser, something she had done a hundred times before. A pain ripped through her hip, shot down her right leg, and froze in her ankle. She couldn't walk. One minute Judith was mobile; the next, she was stretched across the couch writhing in pain. Diagnosed with a ruptured disk with sciatica, her life spiraled into a painful ordeal.

"I tried everything, from epidural injections to physical therapy. The first doctor said I'd have to live with the pain; the second opinion was equally unsatisfying," recalls Judith.

For two years Judith lived in daily pain. Last April she took her last painful step when she entered Dr. James Zucherman's office at St. Mary's Spine Center in San Francisco. He offered her an alternative to her back problem: high-tech spine surgery with a 70 percent chance of success. Judith gambled on success. She won.

Twenty-four hours after her surgery, Judith left the hospital without a stitch. Two weeks later, she was 98 percent pain free, living a normal life and raving about her back surgery. Yes, raving about back surgery!

The Tiny Revolution: Percutaneous Procedures

Judith had minimally noninvasive spine surgery. It may sound like an undercover covert operation, but it's the latest in high-tech spine surgery. Noninvasive spine surgery, the small procedure revolutionizing spinal technology, is performed percutaneously.

Percutaneous procedures go under the skin, but there is no cutting or stitching involved. After a minuscule incision, a straw-type tool, a scope, and in some cases lasers, achieve rapid results. These cutting-edge procedures take between sixty and ninety minutes. Percutaneous procedures are performed on an out-patient basis. Moreover, risk of infection is cut in half and healing time and expense is reduced. If a second surgery is required, the prospect for success remains the same. So with this revolution on the table, why are orthopedic surgeons still performing invasive procedures?

While percutaneous procedures are receiving a lot of favorable press, arthroscopic or endoscopic noninvasive spine surgery is still new to the back field. At present, these techniques are performed only on contained herniated disks that create leg pain. A contained herniated disk means that fragments of the disk have not migrated away from the disk but are still contained in that area. Remember that the spine is a complicated structure composed of separate spool-shaped bones called vertebrae. Sandwiched between each vertebrae is a jellylike pad, or disk, with a center that resembles a jelly donut filling. Stress the disk, and you're in trouble. What we commonly call a slipped disk is actually a disk that has been injured, causing it to bulge or herniate. When this happens the jelly center spurts out. If the jelly stays contained within the disk, a noninvasive procedure is possible. But once the jelly breaks loose and migrates outside the disk, the herniation is no longer contained, and a noninvasive procedure is impossible.

If you have had previous disk surgery, chymopapain, spinal stenosis, a severely ruptured disk, or degenerative problems, you are probably not a candidate for this type of procedure. But if you do qualify, keep in mind that because percutaneous procedures are still in their infancy, it is important that the surgeon performing the surgery have a good track record.

Following are the most promising percutaneous procedures around. They substitute for open surgery, involve a minimum of pain, and are a great savings both in cost and recovery time. Moreover, they are performed under local anesthesia, and the patient goes home that same day.

Automated Percutaneous Lumbar Discectomy (APLD)

Judith had an APLD, an alternative to the most traditional approach to disk removal that was pioneered by the St. Mary's spine surgeon team. It is an automated technique by which the protruding jelly center of the lumbar disk is removed percutaneously by a 2-mm blunt-tipped suction-and-cutting device. Using an X ray picture as a guide, the orthopedic surgeon inserts a nucleotome, a combination suction-and-cutting device, into the center of the protruding disk. The device probes to and fro, loosening the disk material. A pump attached to the probe suctions the material and carries it away. The procedure takes approximately forty-five minutes and requires two weeks' recuperation.

Laser Arthroscopic Microdiscectomy (AMD)

Another alternative approach to surgery is the arthroscopic microdiscectomy, which takes approximately ninety minutes to perform. Like the APLD, the surgeon uses pliable miniature tools that go through a 6-mm cut in the skin. Through a tube, the surgeon winds a thin cable, which carries a tiny video camera to locate the exact spot, to the damaged disk. The cable also transports a laser fiber that vaporizes unwanted disk material. Suction carries the material away. Like the APLD, the surgeon views the procedure's progress on a television monitor as he or she extracts pieces of the hard disk.

Percutaneous Laser Discectomy (PLD)

A laser discectomy entails the percutaneous insertion of a fiber through a thin-gauge needle through which laser energy vaporizes the nucleus or central part of the disk.

Laser spine technology is currently touted as the medical breakthrough of the century. But a word of caution: There is nothing magical about lasers, particularly when it comes to the spine. The location of the nerves so close to the disks makes this procedure precarious if not performed with skill and expertise. Because the surgeon is working in such a small space, great care must be taken to not burn the surrounding tissue and nerves. Again, those people with broken-off pieces of disk, or with histories of previous disk operations or failed chymopapain, spinal stenosis, or chronic degenerative bulging disks are not candidates for this technique.

Vital Statistics and Noninvasive Spine Surgery

Success rate. Minimally invasive surgery carries a slightly reduced success rate than invasive procedures; statistically the success rate is approximately 70 to 75 percent. Some statistics rate success as high as 90 percent with good conservative care. Because no cutting or sewing is involved, potential complications with noninvasive surgery are ten times less likely than with open procedures.

What about a second surgery? Let's face it, no one wants to repeat a surgical procedure. But if you must have a second noninvasive spine procedure, there is some good news. The rate of success does not change with subsequent surgeries. And the comparison between incision and percutaneous procedures is worth noting. While the success rate plummets from 90 to 50 percent with each additional incision, it remains the same with each noninvasive surgery.

Costs. Arthroscopic noninvasive surgery is sometimes as much as one-fourth cheaper than incision-type spine surgery.

In and out in the same day. Percutaneous procedures are done on an out-patient basis. You usually leave the hospital the same day. Because the procedures are done under a local anesthetic, you are awake for the surgery.

Insurance. Check with your insurance prior to having a percutaneous procedure. Some companies still consider these techniques experimental and do not cover them.

The Failed-Back-Surgery Syndrome

Dr. Elterman is hardly a novice to surgery. As a vascular surgeon, he's spent twenty-five years rolling up his sleeves in an operating room. So in 1994, when he was troubled by restrictive pain around his chest, waist, and gluteus, he ordered an MRI and discovered two herniated disks. Opting against surgery, Dr. Elterman struggled with debilitating pain for nearly a year. Unable to stand, he took a leave of absence, consulted with an orthopedic surgeon, and had back surgery in December 1995. The pain worsened and another MRI showed the disk fragment had been pushed upward, irritating the spinal cord. Dr. Elterman got through the next few months taking pain killers. Discouraged, he sought advice from a neurologist. Four months later, Dr. Elterman underwent another failed back surgery. Deperate, and living with constant pain, he has enrolled in a yoga class, sought acupuncture, and continues to pursue a solution. His bigggest complaint, though, is not his pain, but the lack of compassion and understanding shown by his own profession for chronic pain patients.

In almost every case, the person who undergoes spine surgery expects a positive outcome—and the surgeon performing the surgery anticipates the very same outcome. Both hope for a significant reduction in pain, a return to work, and a normal life. Nevertheless, each year 20 to 40 percent of back surgeries will not have the expected outcome. These fall into the category of FBSS, or failed-back-surgery syndrome. In a small percentage of FBSS, the condition may even be worse after the surgery than it was before.

What causes FBSS? Why does it happen to some people and not others? According to Drs. James Zucherman and Jerome Schofferman in a presentation of the pathology of FBSS, only a small number of patients who fail to benefit from lumbar spine surgery will be found to have disorders unrelated to the initial reason for the surgery. The difficult part is discovering why the surgery failed. Possible causes of FBSS can be either structural problems, such as spinal stenosis or recurring disk herniation, postoperative infections, or psychological problems, such as depression or high levels of anxiety. For the individual like Irve, intellectually understanding why a surgery failed doesn't ease the pain and disappointment. For the physician searching for clues to FBSS, the task ahead is a formidable one.

To Cut or Not to Cut

Let's face it, the idea of having back surgery is as appealing as an IRS audit. Nevertheless, the United States performs a whopping number of back surgeries. Surgery for back problems should be your very last resort, only after you've exhausted all other possibilities. All too often, though, as statistics prove, this is not the case. Over 250,000 back surgeries are performed yearly in the United States, costing an estimated $9 million. Furthermore, a third of all surgery requires a second round under the knife. But as mentioned before, with each additional spine surgery, your success rate plummets from 90 percent to 70 percent to 50 percent. For the majority of people who suffer from chronic back pain, then, surgery is not the answer.

Unfortunately, many who suffer from back pain look to surgery as a cure, akin to fixing the plumbing under the kitchen sink. Just take out the injured vertebrae, zap the injured disk, fuse the bones together, and the old back will be as good as new. But surgery cannot always repair mechanical problems caused by wear and tear of the spine.

Remember Hank's chymopapain surgery in chapter 2? It worked splendidly for Hank's back problem, along with a daily dose of exercises. Hank told me that a friend of his who suffered with a herniated disk also had the chymopapain treatment about the same time, and his friend's surgery turned out to be a miserable failure.

How can two people diagnosed with the same back problem have the same surgery and get two opposite results? I could simplify the equation and say it's not unlike two people with strep taking the same antibiotic; one person obtains relief, the other doesn't. But as you already know, the back is much more complicated than a sore throat. Spinal surgery involves more than cutting, stitching, or percutaneous techniques. It involves the surgeon's expertise, and the patient's nerves, mental attitude, and entire body. My body is different than yours, and our aging processes and lifestyles contribute to how we will recover from a back operation, should we make that choice.

If surgery is indicated, familiarize yourself with the types of surgery and *always* seek a second opinion. A good spine surgeon will discuss surgical options and the pros and cons of different types of surgery.

I cannot stress enough, even in the throes of pain, how important it is to take the time to find a good surgeon or spine clinic that specializes in spine care. Look for a spine center that works with a multidisciplinary team of doctors.

TRADITIONAL TYPES OF SURGERY

Spine surgery is rapidly changing. The following surgical techniques have been around for some time. If these are your options, familiarize yourself with them before going under the knife.

Laminectomy

The laminectomy, considered by some the standard of back surgery, has been performed for some thirty years. A laminectomy is a removal of the posterial portion of the ring of bone that surrounds the nervous tissue in the spinal canal. Laminectomies are performed to relieve compression of the spinal cord, caused by a bone displaced due to an injury or resulting from disk degeneration. Performed under general anesthesia, the underlying problem should, theoretically, be corrected. But this doesn't always happen. As with Irve, the laminectomy did not relieve pain, and the problem was not corrected. Sometimes the surgeon does not remove enough of the laminae but has no way of knowing this until after the patient has recovered from surgery.

Fusion

Fusion surgery stabilizes vertebrae that are unstable due to degenerative disks or worn-out facet joints. Fusion is the replacement or bridging across a disk with bone. The bone is either donated or taken from the back of the pelvis. The concept is that living bone will grow over the area in your back and fuse together.

There are many types of fusion surgery. Some techniques involve attaching hardware, such as screws or rods, to the back or front of the spine bones to stabilize them. This surgery is very extensive. St. Mary's Spine Center in San Francisco has recently developed a percutaneous fusion technique that has been successful in over sixty patients at this time.

Microdiscectomy

Microsurgery uses a microscope so that the incision site is only an inch long. This is not a percutaneous procedure, it's major surgery, although pain is less severe than with other dramatic surgeries. Nerves to the spinal muscles aren't cut, ligaments to the spine aren't cut, and tissue damage is reduced. The surgeon's field of vision is more restricted than in a traditional laminectomy. The doctor must be sure of the exact location where the disk is impinging on the nerve; otherwise, symptoms may reappear due to missed parts of the disks. There is less operative pain with a microdiscectomy and more rapid return to daily activity.

Foramenotomy

A foramenotomy is performed to provide a passageway for the spinal nerves from spinal stenosis. The small openings in the vertebrae, called foramen, allow the spinal nerves breathing space. With spinal stenosis, a narrowing of the space within the spinal column causes the nerves to become constricted and swell. With a foramenotomy, the bone around the foramen is shaved, allowing for breathing space for the nerves and blood to circulate freely.

Chymopapain or Chemonucleolysis

Chymopapain, once a controversial treatment, still appears to be in use. With many newer, less invasive surgeries on the horizon, chymopapain has become less popular. Chymopapain, an enzyme derived from the papaya fruit, acts like a meat tenderizer on the nucleus of the herniated disk. It involves partial destruction of the nucleus, as the nucleus of a herniated disk is digested by the injection of chymopapain. The procedure ideally shrinks the protruding area of the disk, thus lessening pressure on the nerve root.

A number of complications plagued chymopapain in the beginning: back spasms, neurological damage, and allergic reactions. As chymopapain's popularity rapidly peaked in the early eighties, many physicians received rapid but inadequate training, underscoring the need for more thorough understanding. Today, chymopapain is skillfully used as a treatment by some doctors. It's less expensive than other procedures and incurs less scarring, but some people are highly allergic to the drug and cannot tolerate it. A preliminary skin test can detect a measure of adverse reaction, but sometimes even the skin test cannot foretell possible problems.

When Spine Surgery Is Absolutely Indicated

If you have sudden loss of bowel, bladder, or nerve control, call your doctor immediately or get to an emergency room. You may be suffering from a longtime injury that has suddenly worsened, cutting off the blood supply from the nerve and killing the nerve cells. Loss of bowel or bladder control indicates possible extensive nerve damage. If not surgically treated immediately, it may result in permanent nerve damage.

WHAT'S NEW ON THE SURGICAL HORIZON

The future of spine surgery may be heading from the back to the front. Laparoscopic procedures are proving successful in certain types of spinal surgical procedures and some percutaneous procedures. Laparoscopic spine surgery may soon be a better and more cost-effective option for spine surgery.

The Bak Implants

The bak spinal implants, still new and not widely available, is used in fusion surgery to stabilize motion in the spine. Bak implants, similar to large, hollow screws with holes in them, are usually implanted in pairs inside the spine. They are made from titanium metal. Bak implants can be put in posteriorly or laparoscopically. They are used to stabilize the spine.

The Pedicle Screws

Pedicle screws are used to stabilize the spine after spinal injury or to correct severe spinal curvatures and other abnormalities. In many cases, they have replaced other methods of spine stabilization, such as wires, rods, and hooks. The controversy surrounding the pedicle screws is that they have not been approved by the FDA but are still widely used. Under the law, before orthopedic screws can be marketed as pedicle screws, their manufacturers must submit scientific data to the FDA establishing that these devices are safe and effective. Limited studies of pedicle screws have been ongoing for a number of years, and the FDA has approved using the screws for the purposes of these studies. According to the April 1993 newsletter of the Back Pain Association of America, the studies on pedicle screws have not been completed and the manufacturers have not accumulated enough data to show, one way or another, whether the screws are safe. Does this mean the pedicle screws are unsafe? Some hold that there is simply not enough scientific data at this point to say one way or the other. Surgeons using pedicle screws believe they are by far the most effective hardware on the market to stabilize the spine, far more effective than the wires once used.

Experimental Surgical Options

Bone morphogenic protein (BMP) is used to help make fusions take and fractures heal. BMP is a protein found in bone that directs undifferentiated cells to become bone cells. The protein signals the body to produce bone at the site where it is found. BMP can now be cloned from other cells who have been engineered to make it, and there are many bone morphogenic proteins with varied potency for bone production. However, BMP is very costly to produce. The "cloned" varieties are still in clinical trials.

A fusion cage is a threaded metallic or cadaver bone hollow cylinder that replaces the inner part of the disk to make the vertebra above and below fuse to each other by attaching to the cylinder. There is hope that these cages will produce better results in cases where a fusion is necessary. The fusion cage is a permanent fixture unless it slips out of position due to unsuccessful fusion.

Last, artificial disks are being developed to save joint motion in people who would otherwise need fusion. There are several prototypes, all of which are experimental at this point. Some problems with artificial disks are loosening, displacement, infection, and delayed deterioration.

Because none of these are tried-and-true procedures, you may want to take a wait-and-see attitude. All these procedures should be inserted by an orthopedist or neuro-surgeon who have been properly trained in the technique.

STAVING OFF BACK SURGERY

You've done everything possible, and like Judith and Hank, surgery is the last alternative for you. Here are a few tips to help you prepare for back surgery and to return to a healthy, productive life after the surgery:

• Search for the right medical team and get a second opinion. Ascertain if the spine surgeon has a pain clinic, a physical therapist, a neurosurgeon, a psychologist, physia-trist, osteopath, or chiropractor on board.

• Ask your surgeon to have the surgery explained to you. Ask about the success rate and risk. Talk about your fears, how you manage pain, and what outcome you expect from the surgery.

• Consider whether your projected outcome is realistic, how much recuperation time is needed away from work and normal activities, and the requirements of your recovery period.

• Discuss with your practitioner what happens if you need another surgery. A second surgery is not so uncommon.

• Follow up with back exercises and changing patterns. Don't expect the surgeon to do any more than perform surgery. It will be up to you to carry on with your back exercises and change lifestyle patterns that undermined your back. Most doctors agree that changing postural habits and exercising can drastically reduce your chances of needing surgery. If you think that you are a candidate for back surgery and are willing to involve yourself in an intense physical workout to avoid that surgery, see the next chapter.

Chapter 11

STABILIZATION

Orthopedic surgeons Arthur H. White and James Zucherman made the medical hall of fame when they operated on San Francisco 49ers quarterback Joe Montana. Fans of the 49ers hailed the surgical feat as nothing less than a miracle when star quarterback Montana returned to the playing field only fifty-five days after his back surgery. There were 200,000 phone calls to White and Zucherman's office the week following Montana's surgery from back sufferers around the country pleading for a chance under their knife.

But the doctors declined. A staunch opponent of back surgery, White offered a more conservative approach, an approach he swears by: stabilization.

"Ninety-three percent of the patients who come to me, all with herniated disks, all put on the surgery schedule in some hospital or another, avoid surgery with stabilization," White says.

White should know. One of the first doctors in the country to specialize solely in spine care, White himself has suffered from a multitude of back problems, including spinal stenosis and spondylolisthesis. But he's never been operated on; he lives and breathes stabilization.

WHAT IS STABILIZATION?

Stabilization is impeccable body mechanics, or relative fixation of the abnormal spinal area that allows it to rest. This approach does not so much recommend maintaining a rigid, impractical lumbar position as much as it recommends, through evaluation and a clear understanding of the individual back problem, an appropriate exercise program designed to train each individual to control and limit unhealthy spinal movement.

Stabilization is a multifaceted program promoting education, flexibility, strength, and endurance to prevent repetitive trauma to the spine. It works on the premise that through a combination of exercises and instruction the individual can stabilize the lower back. It requires work and a great deal of individual participation. While you can learn to do the exercises on your own, it is important that you work with a physical therapist who can teach the principles of stabilizing your movements. Practitioners often speak about lifetime habits of incorrect posture positions, such as thrusting the head forward, slumping over desks, or walking hunched over. Years of these problems—or years of ignoring the spine until one has a serious back injury, such as a bulging disk—cannot be cured overnight.

Essentially, stabilization involves living and moving from one's center, in a way not unlike that of a martial arts practitioner. Once someone is taught to consciously develop the balanced ageless position, as a martial artist does, the aging process of the spine slows down.

Stabilization is a part of many back classes or back schools. It requires a thorough evaluation and ongoing assessment of your back condition. The physical therapist or back class instructor must understand the individual's abilities and problems so that appropriate levels of exercise can be imposed. A good physical therapist should plan a guideline in the form of a hierarchy of skills in order to

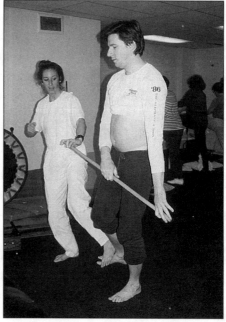

James F. Zucherman, M.D.

provide a good rehabilitation program.

Stabilization typically moves through four stages: *Passive prepositioning* requires minimal muscular effort and is easy and safe for back sufferers. For example, an individual who needs to avoid lumbar flexion would begin the stabilization exercises in a supine position. Something as simple as a hamstring stretch, which depends on the floor to provide spinal stability or a wall that allows the legs to rest, is an example of passive prepositioning. As the lower back improves, the amount of passive exercise may be replaced with *active prepositioning*, which uses muscle activity to correct the spine. An example of active

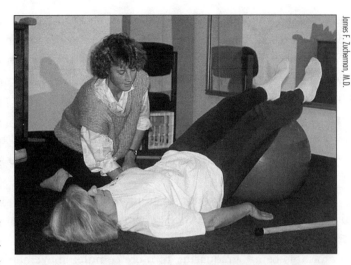

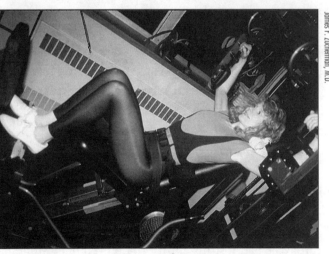

prepositioning is the pelvic tilt, which uses gluteal and abdominal muscles actively. In this stage, the individual can begin to isolate abdominal muscle contraction. At this point he or she uses muscle control to position the pelvis; the body begins to actively engage in the exercise process. The third stage, *dynamic spinal stabilization*, uses neutral or midrange spinal positions. These positions are more difficult and require concentration and control of various muscles. Moreover, the individual must use more than one set of muscles. For example, when you raise the arms overhead, there is a tendency for the lumbar spine to extend, and to counteract this tension a proportionate increase in both gluteal and abdominal muscle contraction occurs. In order to change stress and muscle tension that may take place in this position, one must both concentrate and be aware of the connection between the lower spine, abdominals, and gluteal muscles. Ultimately, the fourth stage called *transitional stabilization* requires a change in the primary muscle movement. It involves a muscle that is opposed by contraction in another muscle, the antagonist. For example, lifting a heavy round ball or object from the floor to waist level requires use of contracting trunk muscles to stabilize. This final stage is often more challenging.

Stabilization must be done on an individual basis with a physical therapist. Exercises must be taught and controlled during sessions. While stabilization progresses from large, easy movements to isolated, complex movements, it is important that you feel comfortable before graduating to more complex movements. According to Dr. White, stabilization must be incorporated into your daily lifestyle to make it work.

Remember, your spine is like your fingerprint, unique and different from that of your neighbors. For some it takes years to obtain good spinal motion after an injury; others are never pain free, and still others jump back into the game immediately.

"I wouldn't recommend returning to the playing field or tennis courts fifty-five days after back surgery," says Dr. White. "In Montana's case, we had worked together for some time prior to surgery."

So why, if Montana had stabilization, did he require back surgery?

Montana had a herniated disk compounded by spinal stenosis. Despite this, according to White, he was able to stave off surgery and throw touchdown after touchdown while working with stabilization exercises. But during a game, Montana blew a disk. When he came to White's office on Monday he was able to do thirty toe raises, but by Saturday he had lost his ability to do even one. Montana had progressive neurological loss, which White says is the only reason to perform immediate surgery. But White claims it wasn't the knife that put Montana back in the game so quickly, it was the stabilization training Montana had already built into his lifestyle.

"Frankly, I would suggest taking it easy after back surgery, but I knew in this case that Montana was safe—he had impeccable body mechanics, and with impeccable body mechanics you can go back to anything in fifty-five days."

As you may have experienced, experts often cannot find the exact cause of your back trouble. This is frustrating for both you and your practitioner, but it means it may be time to consider experimenting with alternative modalities. More and more backache sufferers are turning to less conventional treatments for their back pain. Again, remember: What sometimes proves to be the best alternative method for one back does not always prove best for another.

To the Western mind, steeped in the Cartesian philosophy of mind and body being separate, these alternative treatments are sometimes controversial and can be debated until the sun rises in California and sets in Tokyo. Nevertheless, they've all been around for centuries and are fully embraced in other parts of the globe.

The next part of this book moves into the alternative world of back treatments, commencing with a view of three popular alternative methods used by millions of people in their quest for a healthy back.

PART II

HOW OTHER PRACTITIONERS TREAT BACK PAIN

The philosophy of chiropractics, acupuncture, and yoga each evolved from a culture or tradition much older—and, some would postulate wiser—than ours. Yet each of these healing modalities had great difficulties being accepted by mainstream medicine in this country. Chiropractors were accused of quackery, acupuncturists couldn't get a license in this country until the 1970s, and yoga was considered a fad hippies or eccentrics pursued in the 1960s.

Truth has an odd way of prevailing, but it's usually not without a struggle. Today chiropractors practice in every state both privately and in state-of-the-art spine clinics; and acupuncture clinics and certified acupuncturists are accepted in the treatment for a variety of ailments. Bill Moyers's holistic-health special on public television recently brought acupuncture into our living rooms, giving credence to one of the oldest medical practices in Asia. And yoga . . . well, yoga has finally been warmly embraced by society as a sound form of exercise. Yoga classes grace senior-citizen centers, hospitals, synagogues, churches, universities, spas, gyms, individual homes, and even jails.

Touch is one of the most effective means of healing known to us, and many of the bodywork techniques we are about to discuss involve touch. Others use more subtle, gentle methods of bringing the body and the mind to center.

The wise and the learned know that there are many truths in healing, some overt, others subtle. This section of our book examines the modalities that have tenaciously survived, the ancient medicinal truths that have been brought into contemporary society.

Chapter 12

CHIROPRACTORS

Twenty years ago I lumbered into work, my neck as stiff as a baseball bat. I'd gone to bed the night before feeling great and woke up unable to move my neck. Was it sleeping under an open window, turning wrong in the middle of the night, or just plain voodoo that caused my neck to revolt?

I took a hot shower, applied heat, and smeared on ointment. I went to work hoping no one would notice. I never knew if it was my lopsided posture or the smelly ointment, but one of the architects in the next office suggested I see a chiropractor.

"But I've never been to a chiropractor, and I'm not comfortable seeing just any old chiropractor," I countered.

The architect said he knew of a chiropractor who had been around for a long time and insisted I call him. I did. I explained my situation, and the chiropractor asked me to come in immediately.

The receptionist took a history, then sent me in to see the chiropractor. He talked to me as his hands gently probed my neck and spine. I remember feeling at ease, even though I couldn't move my neck. He didn't take X rays, but kneaded the rock-hard area with a warm, liquid type of heat. Then he had me lie on the table. After positioning the table he massaged my neck, talking all the time, and then, *crack*, repositioned my neck. I felt instant relief, and would have prostrated myself at his feet if he had asked.

Instead, I paid my twenty bucks and went back to work. It never occurred to me that this man would become integral to my health care.

But over the next decade, my neck periodically spasmed, and I would rush in for a treatment. He never asked me to follow a plan of action, such as three treatments a week, or exercise, or stretching. He suggested I pay attention to lifting and that I not carry things on my shoulders. Much later, I traced many of my neck spasms to carrying a heavy suitcase, a stack of books, or a dance bag slung over my shoulder, weighing down one side of my body.

While the field of chiropractics has come into its own, with much more of an emphasis on education and various methods, my own introduction to the chiropractic world was with a wise, old, no-nonsense expert with a very good reputation in the community. He has, alas, long since retired, and as I've aged, my back problems have changed. But I'm lucky to have found another extremely proficient and knowledgeable chiropractor whose techniques, although opposite those of my first practitioner, agree with me, and who almost always eases my backache or neck spasms. I had to search to find her, however, and in the interim I stumbled across a few chiropractors whose techniques or tableside manner did not suit me so well. So be prepared to look around a bit before finding a chiropractor who's right for you.

To help you understand the world and evolution of chiropractics today, let's glance at its history.

Then and Now

Two decades ago, the American Medical Association wouldn't give chiropractors an eye blink. Today, chiropractors are the most widely sought practitioners for alternative back treatment. Chiropractors represent a small but growing segment of health services in the United States. They are members of the third largest group of health care providers after medical doctors and dentists. An estimated two-thirds of all health care visits for low back pain go to chiropractors, and chiropractors are the primary health care providers for about 40 percent of all episodes of back pain due to automobile accidents. So, if traditional medicine doesn't do the trick, you may want to investigate a more holistic approach to treating your back.

Chiropractic care is past the centennial of the first adjustment in 1885. The evolution from an ostracized group of practitioners to an accepted health-care profession is one of the most remarkable social phenomena in American medical history.

In the nineteenth century, orthodox medical practitioners expressed ambivalence about the practice of manipulation—spinal manipulation, as you know, forms the cornerstone of chiropractic practice. Ambivalence gave way to disdain, forcing chiropractors to develop outside the traditional medical establishment.

During the turn of the century many American workers, both rural and industrial, suffered back and neck pain, but at this time no one practiced spinal manipulation. In other parts of the world, however, hands-on treatment by bonesetters, or joint manipulators, had long been a part of even the most primitive cultures.

One family of English bonesetters migrated to New England, and apparently then traveled with their skill to the American frontier. Despite this, bonesetters were rare in the United States. Daniel David Palmer, the father of the chiropractic profession in the United States, may have been influenced by bonesetters. Palmer was, however, greatly influenced by Taylor Still, the founder of osteopathy.

Though Palmer and Still made spinal manipulation therapy available in North America, they were not the first to document the procedure. The first physician to clearly document spinal manipulation techniques was none other than Hippocrates, in his book *On Joints*. There, he discusses two contrasting techniques of spinal manipulation for two types of problems. For the first disorder, scoliotic curves, Hippocrates uses a manipulation procedure called *succession*, a gravity traction administered with force. The second disorder, *subluxation*, in which one or more vertebrae are out of alignment, requires heating the spine and adjusting the individual on a table. The influence of Hippocrates was widespread. Although his method of succession was not widely used, his method of adjusting vertebral subluxations persisted for more than two thousand years.

Today, doctors of chiropractics continue to treat all types of patients with back pain in various parts of the world. And in a recent study last December by the agency for Health Care Policy and Research, chiropractors finally obtained a gleam of long-due glory: In a major departure from traditional practice, federal health officials validated the century-old discipline of chiropractic treatment. Rebuked by the mainstream medical establishment for decades, chiropractics among consumers and the medical establishment have begun to receive credibility.

What to Expect

On your first visit, your chiropractor will question you about your particular problem and discuss the state of your general health. This will be followed by a medical history and a spinal examination. The examination assesses movement and other characteristics related to your spine and joints. Sometimes an X ray is taken to assist in diagnosis and treatment. X rays are useful tools to determine vertebral subluxations and postural problems. They also rule out serious underlying conditions such as fractures and tumors. Depending on the situation, other diagnostic tests may be in order. MRIs are used much less frequently than X rays but are useful when it is necessary to see the inside of the disc or to visualize the internal workings of the nervous system.

Chiropractors do not prescribe drugs or perform surgery. The chiropractic approach works on the theory that the body has inherent healing abilities. Chiropractic care needs no special tools and puts nothing in the body.

According to Michael Gazdar, D.C., C.C.S.P., author of *Taking Your Back to the Future*, the art of delivering chiropractic care has changed very little and while back pain stemming from sprained ligaments and disk disease can be greatly relieved with chiropractic adjustments, referred pain from a diseased organ such as a bad heart or prostate usually cannot. Chiropractors work to restore motion and help relieve pressure around the nerves and roots. Restoring good motion to the joints is the goal of the chiropractor.

Chiropractic techniques are mostly "hands-on" adjustive, manipulative, and physiological procedures. Sometimes ultrasound or muscle stimulation is applied. Because back pain has many different origins, your chiropractor should explain your specific problem. Just as you would ask your physician for a clear statement of treatment, so should you be prepared to do the same with your chiropractor.

From a Chiropractor's Table

Diagnosed with a slight scoliosis as a child, Nadine slept in a body cast at night and spent years in physical therapy. An artist and renowned potter, she hunched over a throwing wheel for years.

"My back ached continually, and I started seeing a chiropractor on a regular basis. Eventually, I had to find someone else to throw the pots; my back couldn't tolerate the hunched-over position."

Nadine gave up throwing pottery and moved into painting for the sake of her back. Her spine recovered, but periodically she needed to see her chiropractor, and she routinely did exercises for her back. The birth of her child left her little time to exercise, but a few months ago she again started horseback riding, a passion she's dabbled in since childhood and one she says strengthens her abdominal muscles. The unexpected fall from her horse hurt her pride more than her back. But the next day all that changed: She couldn't move. Her back spasmed in pain, and she went to bed. Her chiropractor of many years had retired. Did I know anyone? she asked. I sent her to Karen Woodbury, explaining that her technique is vastly different from those of other chiropractors. After seeing Karen six times, twice a week for three weeks, Nadine's vertebrae held in place, and she felt great.

Both Nadine and I had the same reaction to that office, where four chiropractors and a masseuse practice: one of serenity, even with our bum backs. The soothing, gentle ambient music wafting through the background has a calming effect. Karen tells me she was once a stressed-out defense attorney and sought chiropractic treatment after a whiplash injury. So impressed was she with the help she received that she chucked law and returned to school to become a chiropractor. She graduated summa cum laude, specializing in a directional nonforce technique, (D.N.F.T.)

While few of her own patients dive into chiropractics with such intensity, she notes that typically the individuals who see her have back strain or aggravation from a chronic problem resulting from an old injury that never healed. What mystifies most of Karen's patients is why their backs suddenly go out. She explains that something as simple as bending or lifting can trigger a problem, especially if the spine is out of alignment or not strong to begin with.

A lot of people are walking about with misalignment, she notes. Twisting the wrong way can clamp your back into spasms. If Karen suspects trauma, she will request an X ray to rule out a fracture or a tumor. But she seldom demands an X ray unless the patient does not respond to treatment.

An initial visit with Karen consists of a consultation in which a family history is taken. She discusses symptoms and pathology, checks range of motion, and looks for numbness, tingling, reflexes, and loss of sensation. If she suspects a ruptured or bulging disk, she'll request an MRI.

"If a patient has severe pain, weakness, cannot raise the foot, and must alternate between sitting and standing, it may be best to seek another opinion," she says.

Karen's technique uses nonforce—in other words, no rapid cracking or popping. The direct nonforce technique pinpoints misalignments of vertebrae, muscles, and ligaments by using a leg reflex. The same reflex allows for precision in postchecks after the adjustment.

Karen puts her patients facedown on a cushioned table, head peering through a head cradle, and checks for imbalances. She marks all the vertebra, periodically returning to the foot of the table to align the feet. Karen explains that there is a reaction in the vertebrae if they are not aligned properly.

"If you push on the vertebrae toward the right, and it increases irritability, the body reacts by contracting muscles along one side of the body. That contraction pulls the leg up short. If the vertebrae are not misaligned, the feet are even."

Karen scans the vertebrae and pushes on them individually with a light thumb thrust. If the vertebrae are really rotated, or out of alignment, it might take more than one thumb thrust to align them. Through years of experience, Karen can usually tell if the contact between her thumb thrust and the vertebrae works.

Sometimes Karen applies heat or microcurrent, a low level of electrical current, to the painful area, which sometimes helps to speed up the healing process after a treatment. If she feels that a patient might benefit from a massage, it is readily available. Relaxation is part of the healing process. Karen always tries to leave the patient with a positive attitude, something that is not always easy to instill when a person is in pain.

"I tell each individual what to expect and that attitude helps with healing. If the injury is significant, it will take time to heal, and the patient needs to know that."

What Occurs in a Treatment

Spinal adjustment is the key to chiropractic treatment. Just as all physicians do not treat in the same way, neither do all chiropractors practice just one method of adjustment. Essentially, there are many ways to practice chiropractic care, but you can usually distinguish two types of chiropractors: those concerned only with the musculoskeletal system, or back pain, and those primarily concerned with the overall health of the body, including back pain. Whereas Karen uses a nonforce technique, many chiropractors use the standard diversified method. This requires bringing the joints to tension, in which a chiropractor turns or tilts and then gives a quick thrust to the affected area. Where Karen uses a nonforce technique, many chiropractors use the standard diversified method. This requires bringing the joints to tension, in which a chiropractor turns or tilts, and then gives a quick thrust to the affected area.

Remember Hippocrates' discovery of subluxation? Chiropractors use the term *subluxation* to describe the problem that exists when a joint does not function correctly. You will have an assessment of abnormal joint function during your examination. An X ray helps to check for signs of joint degeneration.

Manual adjustment performed by your chiropractor removes the subluxation. This quick, skillful force applied to the body is administered to restore normal joint functioning.

There are several approaches to adjusting the lower back. Minda Dudley, R.N., D.C., uses an activator method. This low-force technique requires a small, hand-held metal instrument that resembles a toothbrush. Using the leg-reflex technique to test muscle tone, Minda lies the patient facedown on a table as she checks for misalignment. Instead of forcefully cracking the joints, Minda puts the instrument over the misaligned area, adjusts the knob to obtain the correct pressure, and pushes it down with her thumb on the vertebrae. The instrument allows her to move from 8 to 40 pounds of pressure, depending on the problem, area of the body, and the person.

"An osteoporatic individual or a person with joint or extremity problems doesn't need a lot of pressure. You wouldn't put 30 pounds of pressure on a joint or fragile bones," says Minda.

Another popular method is Gonstad, a somewhat dogmatic approach to chiropractics. Gonstad practitioners use X rays as a guide for adjustments. They use a lot of rotation to move the bone from point A to point B. Traditionally, the Gonstad practitioner works with a patient several times a week for several weeks, employing not a nonforce technique but rather the diversified method of taking the joint to the end of its range by popping or cracking it.

Tableside Manners

Sometimes you will lie on your side on a table, with the chiropractor standing in front of you to stabilize your shoulders. Other times you may be facedown on a comfortable table. The chiropractor then applies the adjustive procedure to the joints. Another method is placing a small wedge under your pelvis while you lie facedown or up. No matter which way you lie or sit, you should be comfortable.

Will My Back Feel Better after One Treatment?

How rapidly your back recovers depends on the problem. For back pain, feeling better means relief of pain and an ability to resume usual activities. This doesn't necessarily mean the problem plaguing your back has been resolved, however. A degenerative condition or ruptured disk will not be cured by visiting a chiropractor. Yes, the pain may disappear, but the condition may not. One guideline from the Chiropractic Quality Assurance and Practice Parameters is that if your condition is going to respond to chiropractic treatment, it should do so within a one- or two-month period.

Often a chiropractor treats a condition several times a week over a two- to four-week period and then evaluates your progress. If you are uncomfortable with your prognosis, you may need to look elsewhere.

Just as you or I would search for a quality physician, the search for a chiropractor should be conducted in the same way—by word of mouth or recommendation. When I arrived in San Francisco, finding a good chiropractor proved to be a bit tricky. And although I finally found an excellent one, she wasn't the first one I saw.

The first one was recommended by a San Diego chiropractor I respect. And so when my neck spasmed, I called this chiropractor, who graciously saw me at the last minute. He cracked my neck but then started talking about X rays and coming in three to four days a week to align my spinal structure. I objected, explaining that I only wanted my neck adjusted, and I didn't think I could afford to visit him that often. He didn't argue, but I sensed that this was his mode of operation, and I felt uncomfortable with it. I went back home and called everyone I knew who had recently seen a chiropractor, begging for a recommendation. I got plenty, because each person who had found relief through his or her practitioner was particularly loyal. I had the good fortune to find a chiropractor I still see when necessary.

What about Cost and Insurance?

I live in one of the most expensive cities in the country when it comes to health care. My HMO has not yet progressed to include chiropractors. While chiropractors accept insurance, many insurance companies are still in the Dark Ages about covering chiropractic treatment, or may cover only a portion of it. Make no mistake: If you don't have insurance and need long-term treatment, you might have to crack open the piggy bank. I pay $45 a treatment. My chiropractor, after many years of practice, recently raised her rates from $35 a visit. Some chiropractors charge less, others charge more. It is not an outrageous amount of money, but like any alternative treatment that insurance may not cover, the long-term expense can be considerable if you go several times a week.

The good news is that every state offers chiropractic services under worker's compensation programs. Many multidisciplinary clinics with osteopathic physicians, surgeons, and specialists include chiropractors as well. Chiropractic services are covered to some degree under Medicare and Medicaid programs. Many private and self-insured employee insurance programs also offer extended coverage. Today, many chiropractors also have hospital privileges.

TRADITIONAL DOCTOR OR CHIROPRACTOR

Who should you see first when your back revolts? I cannot answer this question for you, and it truly depends on your specific back problem and medical philosophy. Almost every chiropractor I spoke with who suspected a herniated or ruptured disk sent their patients to an orthopedist. If a tumor or other pathology showed up on an MRI or X ray, they invariably sent patients to a specialist. If you feel that you have a grave problem, or if a chiropractor is unable to help you, by all means visit your internist or a specialist. There is no reason for you not to simultaneously see more than one practitioner. As I mentioned in the introduction, beware of any practitioner who believes he or she has all the answers. Ultimately, you have to use your best judgment.

HOW DO I FIND A CHIROPRACTOR?

The best method for choosing a chiropractor? Ask friends or family members for a recommendation. Like any selection process, it may take time; and you may not be comfortable with your first selection. Telephone directories list chiropractic services, but would you choose a physician or dentist by scanning a telephone listing or advertisement? If not, then don't choose your chiropractor in that fashion. And if you are not happy with your first choice, you always have the option to change.

Many alternative practitioners and traditional doctors have a healthy respect for other modalities and sometimes work together through recommendations. Chiropractics is by far the most popular form of treatment in the United States for back problems, but there is an ancient healing art that has been around for centuries: acupuncture. It's been creeping into our Western healing centers, and as you will read in the next chapter, back problems often respond to a few needles.

Chapter 13

ACUPUNCTURE: AN ANCIENT ALTERNATIVE TREATMENT

In 1971, while in China, *New York Times* correspondent James Reston received acupuncture for pain relief after an emergency appendectomy. Reston's rave reviews brought acupuncture out of the framework of Oriental philosophy and into the daily American press. His postoperative treatment was hailed by the Western media. Reston's reporting brought acupuncture into American living rooms at the same time diplomatic doors slid open between China and the United States.

While acupuncture has been a healing art in China for over 3,000 years, its entrance onto foreign soil wasn't easy. Many Western practitioners were admittedly fascinated by the accounts of acupuncture used as an anesthesia and analgesia. But the Chinese philosophy of body dysfunction is very different from the accepted Western view of how the body works. Western medicine is based on the Cartesian philosophy that the body represents one functioning system and the mind another. Chinese medicine assumes the body is a whole and that all parts of it are connected.

Chinese medicine postulates that health is achieved and disease prevented by maintaining the body in a balanced state; thus mental and physical well-being must be combined.

The principle behind the therapy of acupuncture is to balance the body's energy flow. The body is a delicate balance of yin and yang. Yin represents water, quiet, substance, and night; yang represents fire, noise, function, and day. These two opposites must be present to allow the other to exist. Once the vital energy, or chi, is disrupted along any of the body's fourteen meridians or pathways that correspond to primary organs, the acupuncturist corrects the imbalance by putting needles in specific acupunctive points on the body.

When the flow of energy is interrupted, the body's energy unit needs to be tuned up, or balanced. Pain is simply a blockage of this vital energy, not unlike a traffic jam. When your car is stuck in traffic it cannot move, and the energy in your body works on the same principle. Once the chi is blocked, it needs help to circulate. Acupuncture addresses underlying causes dealing with circulation by treating local points. The cause of a problem in your back, for example, may stem from muscle spasms, stress, or a musculoskeletal misalignment. Because everything in the body is connected, acupuncture treats several points. Back pain and neck pain respond well to acupuncture, but while the relief in most cases is immediate, it may not be long lasting. This depends on the problem.

Joy's Story

Joy believes her back might well have been cured from the beginning with acupuncture. She stumbled into an acupuncture clinic after trying several other alternatives.

An active woman, Joy worked from sunup to sundown on a ranch. There were long, arduous hours of climbing, digging and shoveling, and actively keeping her body and mind fit. She's fond of saying that she earned her rest at night and never had trouble sleeping.

An unfortunate disagreement altered the working relationship Joy had with her landlord, so she moved on. For the next year she traveled up and down the state. Her lifestyle altered radically from active to sedentary: sitting, driving, drinking a lot of coffee, and chain-smoking. Bad habits coupled with lack of movement made Joy's back feel tense and stiff.

Joy had a hard time finding work and became depressed. She felt trapped, uptight, and tense. Money scarce, she rented a small room. Lack of exercise and poor eating habits intensified Joy's backaches.

Joy returned to physical work. She began cleaning houses, vacuuming, and rearranging furniture. A compulsive cleaner, Joy went home tired and crawled into bed with a backache. She smoked and drank more coffee than ever before.

Trying to remedy her back problems, Joy tried stretching and back exercises. For a few months she did Pilates, a bodywork program using stretching and machines, but then couldn't afford to stay with it. She moved into a more spacious apartment, but the move created financial stress. By now her back ached constantly.

Fortuitously, Joy picked up the book *Between Heaven and Earth*, by Harriet Beinfield and Efrem Korngold, on acupuncture. It made more sense to her than anything she'd read in a long time.

She decided to give acupuncture a try and without an appointment walked into an acupuncture clinic. Joy credits the acupuncture practitioner with saving her back.

"He put me on a table and put needles in me from my neck to my heels. I fell asleep and dreamed. During the twenty-minute session, the practitioner wandered in and adjusted the needles. I felt completely comfortable, and when I got off the table I was pain free for the first time in months."

Joy continued her acupuncture for nearly three months, combined with Chinese herbs. She credits both the herbs and acupuncture with healing her back and aligning her body. Joy no longer smokes, and she's working toward the day when she will no longer desire caffeine. Back problems, as Joy well understands, are lifestyle issues, and acupuncture treats the whole person, not just the back.

Because back pain stems from a variety of things, most acupuncturists encourage you to check with your doctor to rule out acute problems.

TREATMENT

The sooner the back problem is treated, the faster the condition heals. Acupuncture works best as part of a series of treatments. In China, a series of ten is traditional. Depending on your acupuncturist and particular problem, you might have two or three treatments a week to begin with, tapering off to once a week. It all depends on your condition and how your back responds.

Acupuncture is administered by inserting very fine sterile needles into the body at specific reactive points. You should feel a slight aching sensation after the needle is inserted. This "reaching the chi" plays a role in rebalancing the energies of the body.

If you have ever been treated by an acupuncturist, you may be familiar with a kind of medicinal odor that floats through the office. The odor is not unpleasant and comes from herbs. Herbs are often used in combination with acupuncture treatment. Some acupuncturists send you home with an odd-looking concoction to brew up and drink several times a day. The concoction is typically bitter, and for many, it is difficult to swallow. Herb capsules tend to be a more popular form.

How do herbs affect low back pain? According to acupuncturist and Chinese herbologist Larry Forsberg at the Chinese Medicine Works in San Francisco, herbs are used a great deal in low back pain, because in Chinese medicine other organs, such as the kidneys, are implicated in low back problems. The herbs strengthen the implicated organ. Acupuncture works from the outside in; herbs work from the inside out. Herbs simply build energy, while acupuncture moves energy.

An acupuncture treatment usually lasts from twenty to forty minutes. Needles are placed in the proper points and stimulated. Sometimes the needles are attached to a little box that stimulates the points and enhances the treatment. It is not painful. Sometimes *moxa*, a strong-smelling herblike substance, is used to heat the painful area. The heat is not applied directly on your back; rather, the acupuncturist moves it above the area being treated.

While the prospect of having needles stuck in various meridian points may sound daunting to some, the treatment is actually relaxing. Many people go to sleep or fall into a kind of meditative repose.

Acupuncture is most commonly used for sciatica, menstrual irregularities manifesting in low back pain, muscle spasms, and whiplash.

RISK, COST, AND CERTIFICATION

Acupuncture is not risky, but it can be costly. If your insurance covers acupuncture treatment, you're in luck. If you have to pay for it, it can be expensive. Again, depending on the acupuncturist, the range is approximately $40 to $60 a treatment. I've had treatments for $35, but that was when treatment was recommended two or three times a week. You may want to ask how many treatments your acupuncturist thinks you will need and what the estimated cost will be.

How do you find an acupuncturist? If you are unfamiliar with acupuncture, you may feel more comfortable talking to someone you know who has had acupuncture for back-related pain.

Acupuncturists do not have to be licensed doctors, so you may want to check certification. Certified acupuncturist (C.A.) and licensed acupuncturist (L.Ac.) are nonmedical titles granted by some state licensing boards. Requirements vary from state to state. A diploma of acupuncture (Dipl. Ac.) indicates certification by a national association of acupuncturists. There are over fifty acupuncture schools in this country that certify.

Chapter 14

YOGA

"The approach is so simple and beautiful."

—Mary Pullig Schatz, M.D., author of *Back Care Basics:
A Doctor's Gentle Yoga Program for Back and Neck Pain Relief*

*"In a nationwide survey, chronic back-pain sufferers found yoga
to be the most successful of all approaches to backache relief
for noncapacited backache sufferers."*

—Arthur C. Klein and Dava Sobel, authors of *Backache Relief*

For Dr. Mary Pullig Schatz, back pain was a fact of life. Years of medical school and long hours hunched over a microscope had taken their toll on her spine. Stress invaded her productive lifestyle. As her back pain became chronic, Dr. Schatz recognized the need to manage her stress level, which at this juncture seemed to be controlling her. She began investigating solutions and took a yoga class. To her amazement, her back responded. Dr. Schatz noticed that her back problems were reflective of stress and poor posture.

Doctor Schatz's back problems began in her teens. A tall young woman, she preferred to hunch over rather than tower above her peers. She carried the slouching into her adult life. When Dr. Schatz began practicing yoga she measured 5' 8½". Today she measures a graceful 5' 10".

As Dr. Schatz's posture improved, so did her degenerative back problems. She quit slumping, gave up high heels, and began exercising. Firsthand experience taught her that once the connection is made between lifestyle and a bad back, idiopathic back problems begin to disappear.

As a pathologist plagued by chronic back pain, Dr. Schatz noticed an uncanny thing: Back sufferers came to the hospital for surgery, and within a year or two they returned for another operation. Back surgery often failed because the cause of back problems could not be fixed with surgery.

Convinced that prevention was the key to circumventing surgery, Dr. Schatz began paying closer attention to yoga postures and the effect they had on her back and stress level. In May 1978, Dr. Schatz decided to attend a yoga seminar in Montana. The seminar changed her life, her future, and her career orientation.

During the seminar an Iyengar yoga instructor showed Dr. Schatz how the body and mind are harmonized through yoga postures. In hatha yoga as taught by B.K.S. Iyengar, one develops strength, endurance, and flexibility through body alignment, correct movement, and working with props. Each pose is adjusted to fit an individual's needs. This approach tied together all Dr. Schatz had studied about anatomy and the workings of her own body. Learning how to alter the yoga poses allowed Dr. Schatz to align her body whether standing, sitting, or walking.

The approach seemed so simple that Dr. Schatz took her interest one step further. Rearranging her medical practice, she flew to India to study with Iyengar himself.

Her intent was to learn about musculoskeletal disorders in people with back problems. To her astonishment, she saw B.K.S. Iyengar use yoga for other medical problems as well, such as migraines and high blood pressure. The training was invaluable to her practice. It gave her new insight into how to enhance the body's innate healing capacity using yoga postures and breathing techniques.

Over the next decade Dr. Schatz altered her schedule so that she could spend a month each year studying yoga with B.K.S. Iyengar in India. His approach to altering yoga positions for each person, combined with precision and alignment, energized and inspired the doctor.

Once back in Tennessee, Dr. Schatz began giving yoga classes specifically for back pain sufferers at the hospital. Classes started small; her students were skeptical.

"People with back problems are in a great deal of pain, and this must be addressed before beginning a yoga class. When people are debilitated they feel like victims. They have no control over life and are often angry," notes Dr. Schatz.

Word of her success with yoga for back pain spread. She accepted invitations to travel around the country to speak. She soon discovered everyone seemed to have a back problem, and many were eager for more information regarding yoga and back pain.

According to Dr. Schatz, anytime there is a misalignment in the body, such as rounded shoulders or poor posture, muscles in the back have to work harder than usual. These muscles never get rested, and instead they tense and tighten. When muscles tighten they squeeze off the blood supply. It's a continual negative cycle unless relieved.

By the time back sufferers reach Dr. Schatz's class, they are unable to continue normal activities and are ready to try anything. Most have gone through some form of back school, so her approach is not foreign in encouraging everyone to be involved with his or her own back recovery.

Yoga becomes the medium that allows back sufferers to acknowledge the physical and emotional impact of stress on their backs and their lives. Once this is understood, the body has the opportunity to begin the journey of healing. Yoga is not only therapeutic, it is empowering.

Sixty-five-year-old Adele would agree with Dr. Schatz. Although the two have never met, Adele helicopter skis, bicycles, and practices yoga. A bicycle injury derailed Adele for several months. But after a cervical spinal fusion, she knocked on her yoga instructor, Susan Branum's, door for help.

Branum, who taught anatomy at the National Holistic Institute in Emeryville, California, and who is an orthopedic masseuse and Pilates trainer, has taught yoga for many years. Branum understood that Adele needed to add a little bit of space between the vertebrae; not an easy task after a fusion.

"Adele looked at the swing in my yoga studio and asked what it was for. The hanging-dog pose, I said, as I showed her how bending over the bar of the swing, and letting the head and neck move forward in alignment while keeping the feet against the wall relieves body tension while stretching. When I came back ten minutes later, Adele was still hanging, and she continues to practice on her banister or over a chair," reports Branum, who highly recommends the Hanging-dog pose for stress, tension, or stretching the muscles.

Branum, a one-time modern dancer, turned to orthopedic massage, bodywork, and yoga after realizing that the classical dance stance compromised the spine. Yoga, she claims, is not obsessive or about body image, as dance tends to be. It's rooted in healing, nurturing, and movement within stillness. In her yoga classes, Branum's students move from the breath, and they listen to their body. The individual power resides in the belly, the primordial source of energy. Branum understands that the inner body is what ultimately allows the unfolding of the physical body.

YOGA CLASSES WITH THE BACK IN MIND

Branum's yoga class for the back might seem like an anatomy course at first. Dressed in loose-fitting clothing, her students either lie on the floor, sit in a chair, or stand, depending on the class level and whether pain is chronic or acute. Branum's intent is to have her students feel the spine's natural curves. In the supine position, students lie with backs on the floor and knees elevated, with feet flat on the floor. She works with her students to feel the alignment of the pelvis and to understand how an aligned body feels. Students need to feel the natural curves of their back before they can move ahead.

"I can look at a spine and see scoliosis, or misaligned posture. The thing I must determine is whether an individual uses the body incorrectly or if a structural imbalance is causing the problem," she notes.

Branum claims that since our backside is hidden from view, we neglect that part of our anatomy.

Breathing encompasses the entire body, and in yoga the breath moves through the entire body all the way around to the back. Yoga breathing expands, it's not about limitation. Once the body relaxes through breathing exercises, the class begins with elemental bread-and-butter postures that are good for the back.

The pelvic tilt is the simplest, where you lie on the back, knees up, feet flat on the floor, and subtly isolate and tilt the pelvis to and fro. If her students are able, she follows with a partial bridge posture. Lying on the back, this posture uses the feet and hands to push the stomach upward into an arched position. This does not have to be an extreme movement, and even the subtlest effort stretches the back muscles. Once this is accomplished, students move into the animal poses. The Cat finds you on your hands and knees, resembling a scared cat, hunched up and ready to pounce. But instead of pouncing, the back then concaves, the head moves forward, and the breath is let out. The Dog pose, extrapolated from the Salute to the Sun, which yoga teachers say possesses many of the basic yoga postures in one long series, finds the body with the feet and hands spread apart on the floor, in opposite directions, facedown or stomachdown, thus pulling the hips and pelvis up into the air, stretching the entire torso.

Yoga is always about the quality of the pose, not the quantity. A good instructor works individually with each person, adjusting postures and helping students work through pain. If a yoga posture causes pain, discontinue it or ask the teacher for a modification.

What Is Yoga?

When ancient yogi forefathers devised the perfect fitness program to maintain physical, mental, and emotional well-being, they clearly understood the symbiotic relationship between the body and mind, a bridge Western medicine is only beginning to cross. Through its numerous incarnations, yoga has sprouted an assortment of disciplines and styles. Today, the sophisticated array of postures, movements, and breathing techniques remain a complete science, apt at fine-tuning the mind, body, and back.

Because yoga is an individual discipline, it conjures up different images for different people. True, the five-thousand-year-old practice has its roots in India, but bone-thin swamis posted in the lotus position hardly befit mainstream practice. Modern yoga aims to spirit relaxation and joy into our harried lifestyles by teaching equanimity, flexibility, and concentration.

Yoga is a Sanskrit word that translates into a "perfect method of self-integration or union." When routinely practiced, yoga energizes, harmonizes, and strengthens mind-body awareness. There are several systems of yoga, but hatha yoga is by far the most popular. A physical form, hatha strings together a series of poses called *asanas*. The wellspring of yoga is a breathing technique called *pranayama*. Just as the body depends on water to survive, yoga relies on the breath to move the limbs easily through the poses. Ultimately the *asanas* (postures) and *pranayama* (breathing) render the mind fit for meditation. One pleasant outcome of yoga is the awakening of one's spiritual existence. And, because yoga enhances musculoskeletal strength, flexibility, balance, agility, and coordination, it's a bonus for the back. Yoga takes a holistic approach that a back problem is not isolated from the rest of the body.

Yoga Schools

In response to an endemic interest in fitness and health, yoga's popularity has soared and given rise to a number of yoga schools. Sleuthing through the library of lineages can overwhelm good intentions, particularly if you're experiencing back pain. The following abridged version of yoga schools offers a basic primer for getting started. Classes, instructors, and techniques vary; what does not vary is yoga's goal: to calm the mind and cultivate a state of alert relaxation. If you suffer from back pain when beginning a yoga class, always check with the instructor to see if he or she has expertise in

working with individuals with back pain. I do not recommend one type of yoga practice over another, the following is simply a glimpse of various techniques.

• *Iyengar* pays exacting attention to alignment and anatomical detail. Because of its
precision, Iyengar is a favorite tool for physical therapy and rehabilitation.

• *Integral* combines asanas, breathing, meditation, and chanting into one session. The
classes are flowing and metaphysical. A good place to relax; perfection is not the goal.

• *Sivananda,* like Integral, combines postures, breathing, contemplation, and meditation. Closely related to Integral yoga, Sivananda emphasizes metaphysical practices.

• *Kripalu* favors an introspective approach. Prolonged postures work to release emotional and spiritual blockage. Expect a kindred attitude toward the body and psyche.

• *Viniyoga* has a contemplative flavor with a strong individual emphasis on synchro-
nizing poses with the breath.

• *Kundalini* concentrates on awakening the dormant energy at the base of the spine
by practicing postures, chanting, and traditional breathing techniques.

• *Ashtanga* focuses strongly on the breath through a series of rigorous poses. Expect
to work up a sweat in these classes.

Searching for the Right Yoga Instructor

A knowledgeable yoga instructor is vital if you have back problems. Judith Lasater,
Ph.D., P.T., international yoga instructor and author of *Relax and Renew: Restful Yoga
for Stressful Times,* says yoga is a way of life for instructors. Judith took her first yoga
class at a YMCA in Austin, Texas, over twenty years ago, and she has never been the
same since. "I loved the way yoga made me feel. It felt like I was dancing with the
sacred—a harmonious spiritual and physical alliance. I began practicing daily, and
when my yoga teacher left Austin four months later, I taught the class." Judith's
classes filled to crowd capacity, and she began to think about teaching yoga professionally. There was just one problem, she needed to further her understanding about
how the body worked and find a qualified yoga teacher to teach her the art of yoga. In
retrospect, Judith laughs when she thinks about teaching yoga after practicing for
such a short time. She's adamant about yoga teachers having a certification or plenty

of yoga schooling. Judith's yoga path took her to California where she became a physical therapist and obtained a Ph.D. in East West psychology. "I wanted a more fluid grasp of both the physiology and psychology of yoga to bring to my practice. The practice of yoga is not about flexibility as much as it is about adaptability," says Judith. "The incredible gift yoga offers an individual with back pain is that it teaches them adaptability, something we all strive for in our daily activities. Much of chronic back pain's debilitation centers around stress and poor habitual movements. Yoga slows us down and teaches attentiveness to the body and the mind. It teaches us how to pay attention to our feelings, both inside our body and inside our head. The payoff is that our stress barometer plummets; both our back and body feel better."

Don't be shy about checking out a teacher's background. Ask how many years the instructor has taught and where he or she obtained his or her training, for how long, and whether physiology was a part of the training. Ask if he or she has experience teaching individuals with back pain. If not, it's best to look elsewhere. Just as each back problem is unique, so is each instructor. A good instructor teaches you to pay attention to your own signal of distress, but it is ultimately your own responsibility not to push your body beyond its limits.

Where Does a Beginner Start?

Visit a yoga class and talk to the instructor. If you are practicing yoga to strengthen your back, ask about specific postures. Many exercises prescribed by specialists derive from yoga. And it is vitally important to search out a yoga class or instructor who understands yoga postures specifically designed for back problems. A bad back will not fare well in a class filled with healthy backs.

If there is a yoga institute in your city, call and ask for a referral. *Yoga Journal* magazine (1-800-359-YOGA) offers an extensive directory of instructors, classes, and retreats. For less informal classes, check senior-citizen centers, churches, the YMCA, gyms, and local community centers. A word about yoga videos: There are several good ones on the market, but I have found that videos are not a good way to segue into yoga, particularly with back pain. Nothing can replace the human element of a good teacher.

Chapter 15

A MULTITUDE OF BACK TREATMENTS

Often back pain sufferers turn to bodywork in their search for an alternative practitioner for their particular problem. Sometimes they combine bodywork with traditional modalities of treatment. Bodywork has come into its own over the last two decades, and techniques vary among the different schools.

This chapter discusses the most popular types of bodywork and ancient practices that you may encounter in your search. Rest assured, well-meaning friends who have experienced satisfactory relief from one school will swear that it is the solution to your own back problem as well. It may be, and then again it may not be. Thank them for their gracious concern, gather a few more testimonials, and make your own decision. The differences and similarities among bodywork techniques are subtle; all aim to realign or retrain the body to function naturally. The insightful founders of these healing methods—Feldenkrais, Alexander, and Rolf—each understood that the emotional and nervous system can be organized or rearranged to heal the physical musculature. They believe that the individual has the ability to engage in new learning, no matter how ingrained bad habits are. Sensory re-education is at the heart of several types of bodywork; in other words, you feel it.

This chapter is not meant to promote a particular school of work. It simply offers information on some of the alternatives in dealing with back, posture, and structural problems. Bodywork does not cure a "slipped disk" or "spinal stenosis," but it does help in understanding what may have contributed to spinal problems. Then it goes to work altering ingrained patterns of movement and emotions related to your particular problem. Some of the bodywork and practices discussed have been around for centuries, others for decades. Always seek a practitioner who is licensed, not a student or someone in training.

How expensive is bodywork? That depends with what you compare it. If you compare several bodywork sessions with surgery, the cost is ridiculously low. If you compare it with a session with your chiropractor, the cost is similar or slightly higher. Bodywork traditionally requires more than one session, and ongoing work can be expensive if your insurance does not cover it. Nevertheless, for the individual who benefits from it, or who obtains relief from back or neck pain through a few sessions on a table or mat, the cost is minimal, considering the outcome.

If you are skeptical about bodywork or think it's all hocus-pocus, talk to individuals who have benefited from this approach before you make a final decision. For more information about these methods, see sources listed in the appendix.

Rolfing

Dr. Ida Rolf, a pioneer in bodywork, was a former organic chemist. She perfected the technique of structural integration called Rolfing. According to Dr. Rolf, the traditional idea of standing up straight, shoulders back, stomach in and head high actually misaligns the spine and deforms the skeleton.

Rolf's theory postulates that when the body's structure is corrected, basic chemical changes take place within it that improve overall health.

Rolfing works in ten-session segments. Rolfer and teacher Neal Powers says that's what it takes to take the strain out of the body and put it back in order. The first seven sessions work to make the body strain free, and the last three sessions methodically realign the body along its natural vertical axis. Rolfing straightens the body by correcting the relationship between major body segments (the head, shoulders, thorax, pelvis, and legs) toward vertical alignment. In the last decade, Rolfing techniques have evolved from intense probing to something more akin to sculpting.

Rolfing works with longitudinal alignment of the fibrous tissue, lengthening the body. A Rolfer feels the bundles of irritated tissue and with intense, digging-in pressure, splits the bundles. Similarly, orthopedic massage realigns fibrous tissue, but instead of digging in, orthopedic massage rolls the tissue and allows the bundled tissue to layer apart like an onion.

Rolfers perform deep manipulation of the connective tissue called collagen. The collagen changes from the hands-on energy applied and becomes more pliable.

In a sequence of hands-on manipulation, Rolfers move the tissue back toward symmetry and balance that the body demands. Sufficient force stretches and moves the tissue. Pain may be momentarily intense. Rolfing is not as subtle as other types of bodywork. Sometimes people being Rolfed recall a traumatic episode associated with the body and often emotion is released after or during a Rolfing session. Prices vary from $75 to $120 a session, with $100 the median for an hour-and-a-half session.

MENSENDIECK

Mensendieck is a hundred-year-old paramedical system of correct body mechanics, correct muscle function, and correct posture based on sound fundamental research developed by Dr. Bess Mensendieck. It has widespread popularity in Europe, specifically Denmark, Sweden, Norway, and the Netherlands. Its comprehensive approach and practice is credited in Europe for the low statistics in back surgery.

Dr. Mensendieck was born in 1861 to American parents in New York City. Her father, a civil engineer, traveled extensively with his family. Dr. Mensendieck was gifted both artistically and musically, and made a successful concert debut in Paris before studying sculpture. It was the often awkward bodies of her sculpture models that made her aware of the human form. With a keen eye she began observing children, men, and women. She attended medical lectures on the muscles and finally quit sculpting to attend the University of Zurich to obtain her medical degree. She came to see the musculoskeletal system as a remarkable machine with a marvelous capacity for adapting itself to perform perfectly the most complex movements. She lectured around the continent, explaining her schemes for correcting the common abuses of the body. Dr. Mensendieck set up schools around Europe and in the 1930s opened her first school in the United States.

The Mensendieck system works on the premise that if movements are executed in a beneficial and correct manner, it contributes to a habitually well-functioning body. Mensendieck emphasizes posture and not permitting the skeleton to hang into its frame but to move taller and with natural grace. It is a unique and comprehensive approach, utilizing exercise rehabilitation to address occupational stresses, sports-related injuries, postoperative recovery, as well as chronic back and joint pains produced by bad posture and musculoskeletal diseases. Mensendieck requires no equipment. A session starts by examining one's posture in a mirror. It demands motivation and perseverance to unlearn faulty postural habits, such as slumping in front of the TV, that puts pressure on the sciatic nerve.

ALEXANDER TECHNIQUE

The Alexander technique is a rethinking of how we perform all of our everyday activities, specifically the activities that we take for granted. The educationally based technique is subtle and was founded a century ago by a young Australian actor. Alexander found himself plagued with hoarseness and ultimately laryngitis onstage. Rest restored his voice, but stress weakened it. Alexander reasoned that he must be doing something to cause this. Plotting a course of a discovery, over a three-year period Alexander studied himself while reciting lines. He spent hours in front of a three-way mirror, and found that while speaking he tightened his neck, which caused his head to be pulled back and down into his spine. The result was pressure and strain along the entire back.

Alexander maintains that a person is born with a fundamental pattern of coordination into his or her nervous system. Watch a baby. An infant spontaneously knows when to lift its head, how to sit up, or how to crawl with ease. But as a child grows, he or she begins to imitate the mannerisms of his or her environment, such as parents and peers. A person begins to develop habits such as slouching, slumping, or sitting incorrectly that harm his or her spinal landscape and interfere with natural fundamental coordination. These habits affect muscle development, tension, movement, posture, and breathing and wreak havoc on a healthy spine.

The Alexander technique is a unique method of stopping and changing poor habits. The learning process allows one's sense of coordination to regain the natural balance or perspective. Alexander refers to sessions as lessons and to the patient as the student. It does not involve exercises, psychotherapy, or spiritual healing techniques. Eyes are always open, you are fully clothed, and it's up to the student to pay attention. Alexander believed that in order to produce awareness, the head and neck must be lifted off the spine instead of collapsing into the spine. With this achieved, the neck is freed and the spine lengthens, allowing a completely different manner of movement. The technique essentially looks at posture and how one moves the body in everyday life. Alexander teachers do not follow formal lesson plans. Half of a lesson may be on a table, with the other half taking place while the student goes about a daily activity— playing the flute, washing dishes, or whatever produces the pain.

The technique re-educates people to use their own body in a more efficient way. It is so subtle that one doesn't work to align the mind and body, but must talk to the body and have it listen. Through verbal instruction, demonstration, and light touch, the Alexander technique creates space in the torso. Lessons, tailored to the individual's needs, comprise a minimum of thirty sessions and run between $30 and $55 each. There is no risk to this gentle technique. You'll find variations of it incorporated into back schools across the country. There is a wide variety of Alexander technique teacher-training programs based on diverse interpretations of the technique. Most teachers have completed 1,200 to 1,600 hours of teacher training throughout a three-year period. For more information, see the appendix.

TRAGER®

Peter de Zordo began practicing Trager fourteen years ago. A practitioner at the Trager Institute in Mill Valley, California, he says that Trager is a sensory experience. Trager effects change through passive body movement. It considers body restrictions and patterns of movement. Like several other types of bodywork, Trager is not a confrontive technique.

Milton Trager refers to his bodywork as psychophysical integration and mentastics. Mentastics refers to the mind; and in Trager, the mind is everything. Trager maintains that pain, whether long-lasting or new, causes tension in both the body and mind. Personal or work-related stress, attitudes, and serious health problems impact our daily lives mentally and physically. We are often unaware of how stress affects the mind. The physical body moves on automatic pilot, but the subconscious fear of pain increases tension and contraction in the body. Trager was convinced that the mind holds onto contractions or tension. Therefore, state of the mind is as important in Trager bodywork as is the physical well-being.

Trager was training to be a boxer when he discovered his exceptional ability to work with his hands while rubbing down his trainer. Trager quit boxing to take care of his hands and began the long pursuit that eventually took him to medical school. What distinguishes Tragering from other bodywork is the focus and intent of the practitioner's manipulations.

Trager's focus and intent are not specifically directed toward local conditions in the body tissue, muscles, joints, or skin, like Rolfing, but toward reaching the unconscious mind. It has taken Trager over fifty years to expand and develop his technique.

Trager mentastics is a system of effortless movements to enhance the body's sense of lightness, freedom, and flexibility. Rhythmic massage and stretching movements encourage the body to let go. Through a series of movements—swinging, stretching, pressing, and rocking the entire torso—the body moves into a restful, meditative state. Once the body relaxes, the moves appear effortless. Plan on about an hour to an hour and a half for each session. Trager carries no risk and is gentle. Costs range from $50 to $75 a session, depending on the practitioner.

Feldenkrais

Moshe Feldenkrais, a mind-body holistic health practitioner, was an engineer who worked on the French atomic-research program. A judo master and soccer player, he was forced by an injury to apply his engineering mind to the mechanics of the body and brain. This resulted, in the 1940s, in the Feldenkrais technique. There are literally thousands of exercises in this technique, and the mind and imagination play a key role.

Feldenkrais drew on the works of other pioneers. He recognized that a great deal of pain results from patterns of movement that involve unnecessary muscle tension. Insightfully, he felt people could "learn to learn" to move in a free and graceful way. Feldenkrais held that most people lose the grace, freedom, and joy in movements that they had as infants and small children. He understood that the relationship of movement with thinking, feeling, and sensing can effect changes in behavior, and he coined this "functional integration."

Functional integration may sound like a mouthful, but the subtle exercises communicate to the brain, changing habitual patterns and providing new information to the neuromuscular system by gentle touch, movement variation, and verbal guidance. A movement as subtle as lying on your side, arms stretched in together in front, one palm sliding over the other gently can create an awareness of the upper body and realign movement.

In a Feldenkrais session, a practitioner gently lifts, halts, and supports the head, arms, legs, back, and chest as you are guided through slow easy movements. Touch is light, not deep. Results are instant.

Prior to his death, Feldenkrais worked with individuals affected by multiple sclerosis and cerebral palsy, claiming that his method could improve the health and well-being of anyone having trouble with movement. In some circles he was considered a holistic guru. For Feldenkrais, touch evoked cure.

There is no risk involved with this method. Feldenkrais can be taught in a group setting or individually. Group classes start at around $8, and individual classes may start at $35 and go up from there.

ASTON-PATTERNING

Judith Aston came to Ida Rolf for treatment after an automobile accident. Originally trained as a dancer, she was told she should give up her career. She went on to study Rolfing, but felt that similar results could be achieved with less force. Aston-Patterning postulates that no one has a symmetrical body, that the body is not linear but has curves. Working in a gym on symmetrical Nautalis equipment, for example, works against the body's natural symmetry. So instead of projecting symmetry as the ultimate goal, Aston-Patterning encourages body parts to cooperate with one another through a system of education through movement. Aston-Patterning focuses on three integrated movement systems. An evaluation determines the restrictions limiting movement options; treatment aims at facilitating change throughout the body so that movement is freed up; and the individual performs exercises that loosen patterns of tension. The pace and sequence of Aston-Patterning sessions depends on the individual's need. Aston-Pattering practitioners work with a variety of back and neck problems particularly in individuals who, like Judith, were told they couldn't perform a certain activity again due to injury. The sessions include both massage and movement work, so the client has immediate feedback about how to release tension in the body. Prices range from $75 to $85 a session.

HELLERWORK

Hellerwork is based on the work of Joseph Heller, who also originally trained in Rolfing. He expanded this work to include movement re-education. Hellerwork uses the same deep-tissue manipulations as Rolfing, but also includes verbal interactions that focus on the individual's personality traits and attitudes toward life. Hellerwork emphasizes structural balance and movement education. It also incorporates deep-tissue massage, facial restrictions, postural alignment, and body awareness. Its goal is to realign the body and release chronic tension and stress.

PILATES METHOD

A herniated disk that did not respond to traditional healing modalities resulted in Mathew's exploration of alternative possibilities. He had some success with a healing center, where he was taught to relax his upper body, to breathe, and to practice visualization. And he felt better, but not cured. He contemplated laser surgery, but when the surgeon recommended a more traditional approach, Mathew changed his mind. A pain therapist helped him manage his pain, and then recommended Pilates.

After a few months with his Pilates trainer, religiously taking classes three times a week, Mathew's posture and body mechanics altered radically. He walked differently, and he says his body is more open. More important, today, as he continues to practice Pilates, he feels alive and has few days of back pain.

Introduced in 1923 in New York by Joseph Pilates, this method was the best kept secret of dancers, singers, and movie stars. The late Martha Graham and George Balanchine were some of the first dancers to use Pilates method. Born in Germany in 1880, Joseph Pilates was a frail child dedicated to becoming stronger. He became an accomplished gymnast and boxer. After World War I he studied nursing and designed exercise apparatus for immobilized patients. His designs became the foundation for his style of body conditioning and exercise equipment. Pilates opened his first studio in New York in 1926.

The Pilates method is internationally recognized and has hundreds of certified instructors. Pilates works with muscle resistance in the way muscles are designed to function, not against their natural mechanics. The Pilates method utilizes mental and physical training to teach people how to work from the inside out, to become aware of those deep muscles that you never use in daily activities. Because the method looks at the body as a whole unit, it improves posture, works with breathing, and releases tension.

Pilates method is different from other bodywork in that it uses specifically designed apparatus, which create variable resistance through a set of springs. The apparatus has no relationship to machines in a gym, though the exercises strengthen supporting muscles in the body. Each exercise is designed to stretch and strengthen all the muscles and the joints to release tension.

This holistic method allows each individual to work at his own pace. Classes might work solely with floor exercises which one can practice at home. Most begin with basics such as floor exercises before progressing to the equipment. While each piece of apparatus permits over a dozen different types of exercise movements, several work specifically to strengthen the spine and abdominal muscles. An individual works independently with an instructor, and each program is designed for each person's appropriate physical level. Pilates has become very popular in the last few years. Risk is minimal, with ignorance of how to use the equipment the only potential problem. Pilates can be done in a group or in semiprivate or private classes. Depending on where classes are taken, prices may vary. Typically, a private session can range from $30 to $55, while a twelve-week session of lessons can run between $300 and $500. Prices vary geographically. Private lessons can be expensive. Like most bodywork, Pilates method is done in a series of sessions.

TAI CHI

Many years ago, I watched an elderly Chinese man perform a cross between a graceful dance and a martial art. Fascinated with the slow, meditative movement, I approached the unassuming gentleman, who told me he was practicing tai chi. I learned that he was an ancient master and taught a class on Saturday morning in the park. I joined the class and later studied privately with him. Although I admired the beauty of the movements,

I couldn't seem to concentrate and found my mind soaring above the trees. I quit, and through the years, as tai chi's popularity grew, I noticed individuals practicing tai chi on the beach or in parks, and hoped that at another time I might be a more attentive student. Twenty years later, in another time and place, tai chi reappeared in my life.

Authoring a book is stressful. Sitting at a computer screen or in the library challenges one's back, eyesight, and head. Halfway through this book, I realized I badly needed to balance my stress and confinement at the computer. I returned to the graceful martial art of my youth and began tai chi class one night a week. I marveled at how relaxed I felt after the first few sessions.

One of the oldest martial arts, tai chi is also considered the mother of the martial arts. Tai chi was designed to make manifest the *I Ching*, or *Book of Changes*. No one knows who wrote the *I Ching*, but the ancient book declares that everything in nature houses a yin and yang, two energies that are found everywhere in the universe. Originally, the book was used as a meditation tool and to predict the future, but the philosophy was later developed into movement, or tai chi. Tai chi charges that everything in nature shows the balance of two energies. Tai chi uses the names of animals to describe the movements and their relationship to the universe. A movement like the Crane reflects the yin, or retreating and less substantial energy, while Carry the Tiger to the Mountain reflects the yang, or strong, forceful, forward energy.

Both nature and the self, like a life force, consist of both energies. Tai chi holds that bringing these two energies into harmony benefits one's health both mentally and physically.

Tai chi originated centuries ago in China to improve endurance, flexibility, and balance. The tai chi practitioner understands that human beings are constantly changing and always working through inner conflict. Change is a given in life; tai chi helps you find a balance in that change. It does so by reducing stress, preserving youth, and enhancing good health. Tai chi is an internal martial art, internal because it is based on working inside one's system, the mind and body. With the mind, tai chi controls our thoughts: inside the body, it works to control our energy, or chi. Tai chi is a top-down method. It connects the mind at the top to the body at the bottom. It works simultaneously on the mind, body, and chi.

To practice tai chi, you must become aware of your body and how you move. You cannot practice tai chi without first becoming conscious of your physical presence.

Because most of us use our body incorrectly, tai chi works with warm-up exercises to acquaint us with how the body should function in movement. Hip rotation and waist and arm rotations warm the body. Tai chi rotates all the joints in the body. Chinese medicine believes that if the energy is static or blocked in the joints, aging ensues. When the joints open, one feels better, and the aging process is slowed. Tai chi is a gentle martial art that must be practiced in order to experience the benefits.

This graceful discipline is as reflective as it is vigorous. The effect is one of relaxation and pleasure. I think of tai chi as the universe in harmony. As we constantly change and shift, we must learn to balance life, and tai chi is the guardian of that balance. It is also a good exercise for the back in that it requires a therapeutic routine in which the mind and body must move together to maintain that fragile balancing we all strive for. There is little risk involved with tai chi. Cost varies, but classes range from $8 to $10, perhaps higher in some cities. Group sessions may be cheaper, private sessions more expensive. Tai chi can be practiced anywhere, inside or outside.

REIKI

While visiting a spa in northern California, I stumbled across the Reiki technique quite by accident. I was hiking and discussing back pain with a couple from San Francisco who told me that their daughter had suffered from terrible back trauma. A few sessions with a Reiki practitioner had cured her back problems. I had never heard of Reiki but decided to seek out a Reiki therapist and made an appointment for a session at the spa. The practitioner combined Reiki, a kind of laying of the hands on a person, with reflexology. She explained that people sometimes feel an incredible sense of release, like a bubble bursting, during a session. These releases can cause an individual to cry or feel emotional after a session. This is how the couple had described their daughter's experience.

While my Reiki session was divinely relaxing, I did not have the same experience as the young woman who felt cured from back pain with Reiki. What I did notice is that the practitioner picked up other troubled spots in my body with the gentle movement of her hands. And I nearly fell asleep on the table, feeling like a relaxed noodle when the hour session was finished. Perhaps something subtle was released but I was too relaxed to notice.

Reiki is relatively new in the United States. Its ancient roots trace back to Japan. *Rei* refers to the universal and *ki* the life force or energy. Reiki may or may not cure whatever ails you but it will certainly relax any stress running amok in your back.

Meridian-Based Therapies

Traditional Chinese medicine is a unified healing system that has evolved over the past 3,000 years. It covers acupuncture, herbal therapy, massage, exercise, and diet. In traditional Chinese medicine, prevention and treatment of disease is stressed by strengthening the body's own self-regulation, thus restoring the body's balance within.

Chinese medicine postulates that the life energy—chi, or ki—flows along invisible body pathways called meridians. The chi is the life force that circulates through the body, and its balance is considered to be the essence of health. When the chi becomes blocked at specific pressure points, illness occurs. The following are a few approaches, based on acupressure/finger pressure, to unclog the energy paths by manipulating the pressure points, thus balancing the body.

Acupressure

Acupressure, an ancient therapy for tension and pain relief, uses the same points as acupuncture. The distinction between acupressure and acupuncture is that needles are used in acupuncture, and a gentle but firm pressure of the hands is the basis for acupressure. Acupressure is the older of the two techniques. Acupressurists postulate that the power and sensitivity of the human hand is most effective in relieving tension related to ailments. In order to relax muscular tension and balance the vital forces of the body, acupressure uses a system of points. Acupressure sessions focus not only on relieving discomfort but on responding to these tensions and toxicities in the body before they develop into an illness. The practice of acupressure has developed primarily through a combination of instinct and hands-on experience. A session runs between $20 and $30 and incurs no risk.

Shiatsu

This method of finger pressure has been used widely in Japan for over a thousand years. During the Tokugawa period in Japan, the shogunate organized a school of massage for the blind in order to give them a profession. From that time until World War II, *anma*, or Japanese massage, was practiced primarily by the blind. These blind professionals were known as *anma-san*. They walked through the streets blowing high-pitched bamboo whistles to alert their clients that they were available to come into their homes to give a shiatsu treatment.

Today the shiatsu practitioner, often a small individual, uses his or her palms, thumbs, feet, and sometimes knees to apply a rhythmic pressure to the body. By using finger pressure on the acupuncture points, shiatsu stimulates the chi to flow through the bones, nerves, arteries, and skin. Moderate pressure applied all over the body stimulates the flow of energy. While there may be moments of intense pressure, shiatsu promotes a feeling of well-being and relaxation. The environment is relaxing and peaceful. Shiatsu can help your backache by stimulating your life-blood energy to flow.

While shiatsu applied correctly has little risk, some folks don't care for the intense pressure. There can be moments where the pressure borders on pain, but once released, the pain gives way to relief. Ask your practitioner to adjust the finger pressure if it is too intense. Shiatsu may not be as relaxing as a Swedish massage, which uses stroking movements, but the result is one of rejuvenation and balance. An hour shiatsu session costs between $50 and $60, and it ends with a cupped pounding on the back to wake up the energy. Truly, you feel reborn after a shiatsu massage.

Reflexology

Reflexology is a Western pressure point therapy that focuses on the feet. It asserts that our feet truly connect us with the earth. Our feet are our foundation, yet we remain unaware of them. Reflexology holds that points on the bottom of the feet are linked to specific organs. By massaging these areas, health is promoted to corresponding organs. Reflexologists believe that toxic deposits collect in the feet and that reflexology breaks them up and facilitates other parts of the body.

If you are interested in more information on bodywork, check the list of resources and information in the appendix.

Since alternative bodywork has been refined to an art over many years, you may find components of these techniques in back schools around the country. If your physician directs you toward a conservative approach for treatment, back school will certainly be included. The following chapter doesn't cover the whole curriculum when it comes to back schools in this country, but it does give a perspective on how back education helps you.

Chapter 16

BACK TO SCHOOL

Mark stretches on his back on his living room floor, one leg extended, the other parallel against the floor. His back is flush against the carpet, his hands grip the two opposing ends of a long rubber material that cradle the extended foot, and with the intensity of a sports fanatic he breathes, holds the position, and alternates legs. Then he flips through a "Back School Exercises" brochure and flops over onto his stomach, proceeds to lift his head like a cobra, and stretches his thoracic spine. He holds the posture and in slow descending motion, drops his head to the floor. He continues a series of exercises for twenty minutes. He swears he'll do them every day.

It's odd to watch this 6'2" hulk of a man perform subtle back exercises. But years on the baseball field, running triathlons, and golfing have left Mark with severe back pain at forty-four years old. He's hoping back school will allow him a few more good games on the golf course.

WHAT IS A BACK SCHOOL?

In his book, *Back School and Other Conservative Approaches to Low Back Pain*, Arthur H. White writes, "Back school is insurance against reinjuring your back, providing a comprehensive approach to your back problems. It is an educational training facility that teaches back health care and body mechanics to enable the individual to return to normal activity and avoid further back pain.

Back schools require participation. Like learning a new dance, you can't sit on the sidelines and get it; you must participate. Through participation you obtain a clear understanding of what contributes to your problem. Back school is work, but in the long run, if you expect to have a healthy spine, you'll realize that all that work pays off.

Like orthopedic spine care, back education is a fairly new phenomenon. It did not begin in this country, but in Scandinavia. In America, some specialists began educating their patients about their back problems long before back schools became popular, but the concept of back pain being relieved with back education isn't so very old.

Back school in this country can be traced to Dr. Henry Fahrni, who in 1958 began helping his back patients by educating them about their back problems. Dr. Fahrni recognized the difference between ground-dwelling and industrialized cultures and their relationship to back pain. He concluded that ground-dwelling cultures, or those cultures that squat, developed disk disease in the fifth and sixth decades of life instead of the third decade of life, when degenerative disk changes begin to occur in our spines.

In the late sixties and early seventies, Scandinavians began experimenting with industrial back education. The Volvo factory in Sweden successfully developed a group educational approach for employees who had spine problems.

In 1976, Dr. Arthur H. White and William Maitmiller, R.P.T., opened a revolutionary back school in San Francisco. Their goal was to make back school part of the daily vocabulary of orthopedic care. Their approach to back school followed strict yet unorthodox guidelines. Keep it simple, inexpensive, no hands on, no heat, no ice— just education. This forms the cornerstone to patient education in other spine centers across the country as well.

Back Education Today

Back schools may be part of either a hospital or industrial or specialized spine-care center. You may need a referral from your physician to enter back school in a medical environment. The goal of a back school is to help in the recovery from pain in a variety of ways. A back school in a hospital may be different from a freestanding spine specialty clinic, like the Texas Back Institute or the Florida Back Institute, although the goals are the same.

At Kaiser Permanente in San Francisco, anyone can go to the spine clinic. The group sessions are divided into three meetings: The first class entails a lecture that includes anatomy, physiology, and discussion on how the back is easily injured. The second teaches stretching, muscle awareness, and reconditioning. The third class works directly with stabilization, using objects like Swedish balls and free weights.

Richard Aptaker, D.O., and chief of the Department of Physical Medicine and director of the San Francisco Spine Clinic at Kaiser Permanente, says the emphasis must always be on teaching the patient to care for his or her back problems in daily situations. But Aptaker also understands that back pain is not isolated from the emotional traumas steering the course of one's life. Trained as an osteopath, he treats the whole individual, not just the back. A sympathetic ear and a box of Kleenex are sometimes as relevant as medication, he notes.

A trip to Kaiser Permanente's back class doesn't always do the trick. For the individual who has undergone physical therapy and still suffers from a painful back malady, Kaiser Permanente offers an intense spine-conditioning course.

The eight sessions meet over four weeks for two hours. Ultrasound, traction machines, exercise, and discussion are all part of the sessions. Like its sister spine clinic, it's a communal effort. Trained specialists, however, continually work with each individual to further his or her understanding and education about the back. While many hospitals around the country offer back classes, they are not necessarily state-of-the-art spine clinics.

BACK INSTITUTES

If your back problem cannot be treated by your local physician, you may choose to seek out more specialized care at a back institute. Major back institutes have board-certified specialists who work with the individual to successfully conquer back pain and break the cycle of disability. Diagnostic tests help your physician evaluate your problem and recommend a course of treatment.

Physical therapy plays an important role in recovering from back problems. What I may refer to as back schools many institutions call generalized P.T., or generalized physical therapy, taught by physical therapists. These educational classes may integrate several different programs. Some may be taught in a group setting; others, privately. Miscellaneous exercises, including range-of-motion, bending, and twisting motions, may be integrated into the program as well. Some stretching and general calisthenics may be a part of the school. Isometric exercises, which require holding and contracting, are used to strengthen muscles. One popular program is the McKenzie program, developed by physical therapist Robin McKenzie, founder of the McKenzie Institute in New Zealand, in which the individual moves through a variety of movements that include flexion, lateral bending, rotation, and extension. As I mentioned before, ancient practices such as yoga postures and some types of bodywork have in some fashion been incorporated into back classes. Physical therapy encourages the individual to play an active role in the recuperation process.

Whether attending back school at your HMO or at a high-tech spine center, school requires your learning what caused your back problem in the first place. Generally, back schools cover the following topics: anatomy of the spine, body mechanics, relaxation techniques, and first aid for back injuries. You should always receive a back owner's manual that includes information on how to work, sit, and play sports with the optimum understanding of how each activity affects your spine. You learn how the spine and the entire body function as a whole unit. Think about it: Your back is the largest portion of your body; it's connected to your head, arms, abdomen, and legs. Nerves run through your spinal canal that affect and stimulate your entire torso. Back education today not only touches upon lifestyle changes to prevent painful recurrence of back episodes, but focuses on maintaining the whole body.

One of the most important factors about back school is the emotional support and understanding you get about your specific problem. Because back pain is so darn mysterious, exasperating, and difficult for someone who has never suffered a debilitating episode to understand, often you, the back sufferer, get very little emotional or psychological support from family, friends, or coworkers. Back pain can be an isolating journey. No one need travel it alone.

WHAT IS THE BACK SCHOOL SETTING LIKE?

Back schools or generalized P.T. may vary among settings, but they traditionally offer practical advice, and a kind of back group therapy, with experts guiding, advising, and giving emotional support. Not all back schools are the same.

A back school is an institute of healing. The staff is there to help you heal. Freestanding back schools generally consist of physicians; orthopedists; neurologists; rehabilitation experts such as physical therapists, who have knowledge and expertise in back care and preventing injuries; therapists; radiologists; occupational therapists; and anesthesiologists. Your lifestyle and individual concerns must always be addressed.

While it may not always work for everyone, back school is an excellent approach to heading off expensive treatment, hospitalization, and surgery. Your back-education environment should also offer follow-up courses and refresher sessions as needed.

The YMCA offers back-care classes at various centers around the country. These may not be as extensive as back schools attached to hospitals and spine-care centers, but they do offer a less costly alternative and teach good body mechanics and posture.

GOALS

Once the patient is evaluated, the back school sets a written goal or plan. These goals need to be discussed. In a study conducted by Dr. Richard Deyo, professor of internal medicine and health services at the University of Washington, it was found that patients with back pain do not always obtain an adequate explanation of their problem. The key to breaking the chain of back pain is old-fashioned education. Back school can and should be an institution of enlightenment.

Another goal is to teach the individual simple relaxation techniques and meditation. Keeping a journal of related events that ignite back pain is useful. No one will kick you out of back school if you don't keep a journal, but tracking events that create back pain helps your therapist better evaluate your condition. It's also a great lesson in responsibility.

Teaching general health is vital in back school. The deleterious effects of obesity cannot be overstated. While good nutrition does not always dictate weight loss, obesity must be addressed in back pain. Back school offers counseling in the arena of weight loss, nutrition, and such detrimental habits as smoking.

Another goal of back school is to help you avoid invasive procedures such as surgery. When back school fails to heal your back problem, an invasive procedure may be required, but this does not mean that the back education you obtained in school should be tossed out the window. Embrace what you have learned, and incorporate it into your daily practice. Remember, surgery is no replacement for good spinal care.

If back school is a success, it serves society by reducing the cost of back care and allowing you to return to a normal, productive life.

HOW DO I FIND A BACK SCHOOL?

Many hospitals have back schools or may be able to refer you to a spine center. Ask your doctor for a recommendation, or look in the yellow pages for listings under Generalized P.T., Spine Care Centers, Back Schools, or Physical Therapists.

Check the appendix of this book for some of the top-rated back schools. The listings are not endorsements of back institutes or spine-care centers, but are there to provide good sources of information on back problems, back education, and referrals in your area.

The final part of this book journeys through the uncharted territory of prevention. No, prevention is not new, it has been around for centuries; we simply haven't valued it. But preventive measures offer valuable insight into the insidious back attack and can allow the back pain sufferer to finish a tennis match or end a long day at the desk, pain free. Prevention is finally coming out of the closet and into the medical establishment.

Part III

PREVENTION

The origin of the verb *prevent* derives from the Latin *praevenire*; *prae* means "before" and *venire* means "to come." Prevention is the noun, the safeguard to a healthy mind and body.

In spine care, prevention is both cheaper and simpler than cure. Our traditional reliance on cure has been costly both to the health-care industry and to our own health.

We must ask ourselves: Have we created obstacles on the road to prevention, or simply chosen to ignore the road signs warning us of impending disasters? In the case of back pain, I believe most cases are preventable, particularly if back education begins in childhood.

If you already suffer from back pain, don't give up on preventive measures. Prevention starts by unraveling a lifetime of bad habits. All too often, prevention does not play a role in back care until the onslaught of pain.

Part III of this book acknowledges simple patterns in our daily lives that can transform our back problems. From pattern awareness, the section moves through basic reflective practices and easy remedies for a back attack. A chapter on exercise, the best form of health-care prevention, discusses how a particular sport can affect your back. Ultimately, the book concludes with a plug and praise for ergonomics, the study of equipment designed to reduce discomfort.

Let's begin by looking in the mirror at our posture.

Chapter 17

SELF-CARE:
AN ABSOLUTE NECESSITY

An ounce of prevention is worth a pound of cure. The age-old adage couldn't be truer when it comes to back pain. Back pain is not about cure, it's about care. No matter how much money you spend on treatment or technology, the best way to maintain a healthy back is through low-maintenance, cost-effective prevention. The goal of this chapter is to chart ways to nurture your back in the course of daily life activities. Let's face it, the average lifestyle is incompatible with a healthy back. So whatever treatment you seek, take the time to re-educate yourself about your back. Start with basics, take a look in the mirror.

POSTURE

What do you see when you look in the mirror? How do you hold your body? Are you lopsided? Are your shoulders slumped or rounded? Does your chest concave? Are you swayback? Do you stand like a soldier awaiting inspection? Does your chin jut forward? Does your stomach drape over your belt? Do you slouch on one leg? Did you know that posture reflects self-image?

An array of our back problems can be traced to poor postural habits. Posture isn't just standing; it is the way you sit, the way you carry objects, and the way you move, even the way you sleep. You cannot escape posture; you carry it everywhere.

Walking with a heavy purse or pack of books slung over one shoulder creates curvature problems in the spine. Slumping in a chair in front of your favorite basketball game puts pressure on your sciatic nerve, working at a computer with your shoulders slumped forward creates tremendous neck and shoulder strain, and if you pick your baby up off the floor, while bending at the waist with locked knees, this stresses the lower back and neck. Take a moment to reflect on a few of your daily activities. Are you a sloucher or intent on lunging toward that computer screen? Do you sit in a rolled-up couch-potato position while watching television? Throughout our lives and our daily activities we jeopardize our backs. Prolonged postural imbalance ultimately leads to more serious degenerative problems later in life.

Where Do We Learn Poor Postural Habits?

Watch a family stroll down the street together. Do you notice any similarities in their gait? Their posture and manner of walking is most likely the same. Maybe they swing their arms, maybe their shoulders are rounded or their head lowered. Even if you have inherited poor postural traits, the good news is that you can correct poor posture once you make a conscientious stand to do so.

STANDING

Perhaps you were taught to stand up straight, chest out, shoulders back. The military stand is not a natural one and can give rise to a weak back. This posture allows the forward curve in the lower back to accentuate, leading to swayback. Swayback places stress on the intervertebral disks, particularly in the lumbar area. Stress in this area can cause herniation and sciatic pain. Swayback is a significant problem found in the way people stand.

How should you stand? Do by all means stand tall, throw your chest up and out, and pull in your abdominal muscles. Keep your chin down, and don't let your stomach slouch. Keep your hips and pelvis tilted slightly forward. Allow a tiny curve in your lower spine. This keeps excess pressure from being placed on your lumbar vertebrae. Distributing your weight uniformly along your spinal column helps prevent weak areas from being stressed. Taking bodywork classes or working with a bodywork instructor is an excellent way to realign your posture.

An Instant Posture Test

Stand with your heels, buttocks, shoulders, and head against a wall. If you have space between the wall and your lower back, you have too much swayback. Shuffle your feet forward. This allows the back to move down the wall. Rotate your pelvis backward and tighten your abdominals. Slide back up the wall into a new position. The space between your lower back and the wall should be much smaller than before.

Now that you are on the road to good posture, what else could possibly throw your back out of line? Several things, and although you have no doubt read and heard the litany before, here's the lecture one more time.

Obesity

Do not underestimate the role obesity plays in damaging your spine. A potbelly is a definite detriment to a healthy back. Not only does the excess weight pull you out of balance, but your abdominal muscles are too weak to support your lower back.

Shedding pounds takes a load off your back. Sounds simple: Just drop a few pounds and tighten your belt. But if you have a history of struggling with weight problems, you know that dieting is no simple proposition. Losing weight to help your back requires a long-term change of eating habits and exercise. It is a lifetime commitment that won't happen overnight—nor should it.

Choose a healthy diet, with food that nourishes your body. Talk to a nutritionist, a doctor, or join a weight-loss group. And exercise, exercise, exercise.

Smoking

What does smoking have to do with a bad back? Plenty, according to the latest on smoking and back recovery. Smoking reduces the nutrients carried to the disks in the spinal column. Smoking is bad for your health and your back. Some researchers believe that a cigarette smoker's cough can put pressure on the disks, causing pain.

Beds and Mattresses

Sleeping doesn't have to be a pain in the back. What are you sleeping on? Is your mattress lumpy? Does it sag in the middle, or is it a piece of foam?

You don't have to spend a fortune on a good mattress. Experts agree that a firm mattress is best. Don't neglect a good, firm mattress because you use it only for sleeping. If you cannot afford a new mattress, try putting a piece of plywood board under your current mattress, or putting your mattress on the floor.

Many people sleep on Japanese futons, which can either be placed on the floor or on a frame. Ultimately, the best way to select a good mattress is to shop around and try out different ones. Don't be talked into the first mattress. Try several, and select what feels best for you.

Sleeping positions can create painful spinal problems. Don't sleep on your stomach. Do sleep on your back. If you have chronic back problems, try putting a pillow under your knees. Sleep on your side, bringing your knees toward your chest. Don't sleep with a lot of pillows stuffed under your head.

EXERCISE

Did you know that exercise is the single most important thing you can do for a healthy spine? Many of us slow down physically in our early forties or after we have families. This is not the time to sit on the sidelines. Regular exercise maintains good muscle tone, circulation, and mobility, all of which deteriorate rapidly without exercise as we age.

If you already have a serious back problem, don't choose a strenuous sport. Do find an activity like recreational swimming or walking that is easy on your back but that activates circulation and gets those muscles pumping. The more you exercise, the better you will feel. I promise.

Stretching

Don't jump on the tennis courts or take off jogging without stretching. As a matter of fact, don't do any type of exercise without warming up with a stretching program. While stretching should always be a prelude to a sporting activity, it's a wonderful way to maintain your back and body without actually participating in a sport. Stretching helps your muscles maintain flexibility. Stretching lengthens the muscles.

Take a few minutes before bed or upon rising—even though your body is probably not at its most limber in the morning—to stretch. Now, there is a way to stretch, and bouncing, like you often see athletes doing on the playing field, is not the way. Don't bounce. Bouncing can result in muscle tears and tendon problems. Bouncing causes your muscles to become tighter, not looser. Gently stretch, and hold your stretch for at least fifteen to thirty or forty-five seconds. Do not hold a stretch that is painful for your back. Gently and slowly move into a stretch. If you have not stretched or your body is not flexible, go slowly. Don't expect to touch your toes on Friday if you can barely bend over on Monday. Obtaining flexibility is an act of time and patience. I like to spend a few minutes each night winding down with some gentle stretching.

Sitting

Sitting is an unhealthy occupation for a sore back. It's also very painful for anyone with disk disease. In my chapter on ergonomics, I will cover the proper way to sit and appropriate office accoutrements. If you are engaged in a sedentary occupation, take as many breaks as possible, and stretch instead of gulping a cup of coffee.

Lifting

I discussed lifting in chapter 2. So again: When lifting, always bend the knees; do not bend at the waist. Let your leg muscles do the work, not your back muscles. Never bend without using your legs.

Think about what you are lifting. Before you offer to help your brother-in-law move his refrigerator and washer and dryer into his new house, make sure you have enough muscle power. Better to be a wimp than have a bad back.

Sex

Having sex with a sore back is definitely not a pleasurable experience. But for someone with chronic back problems, sex can often be painful, and ultimately undesirable.

Psychologically, your sex life can take a permanent dive with a bad back. Your partner may not understand your back condition, or the pain involved with movement. Communicating your needs is vitally important to maintaining a sexual relationship during a bout of chronic back pain.

There are various sexual positions that may work for you. Discuss them with your doctor or physical therapist.

Ask about positions that you should avoid that can put stress on your back.

Housekeeping

Did you ever stop and think about your back when washing dishes or preparing a meal? If you are standing over the sink or cutting board in three-inch high heels, you most likely have to hunch over or tower over your work space. Don't be surprised if your back begins to hurt. Make sure that your working space is at the appropriate level for you to cut, chop, and wash. Also be careful when reaching for a bottle of catsup on the top shelf of your cupboard. This is not the best time to practice stretching; use a step stool.

Vacuuming, that undesirable, all-American activity, can be painful with back problems. Vacuums were definitely not engineered by a housewife who understood the ins and outs of vacuuming, or by anyone who knew about orthopedics. Don't huddle over the vacuum cleaner. If your vacuum handle doesn't allow you to stand up straight, bend down on one knee to get into those dirty corners. Don't vacuum for long periods of time. If you are having back pain, either find someone else to do the vacuuming or live with the dirt.

Finally, stay away from stuck windows if you have a bad back. Don't try and open a stuck window, no matter how strong you are. This is the quickest way to strain your back. Ask for help if a window does not glide open.

THE PSYCHOLOGY OF PREVENTION

When we are emotionally tense, we secrete excessive adrenaline into our muscles, causing them to tighten up. I have found an interesting correlation with my back problems and my life. Whenever my back goes out, it always coincides with stress or stressful passages. Sometimes I'm doing too many things too quickly; I'm not centered, and it's always my back that acts up.

One friend told me that whenever she has to make an important decision, her back goes out. She relates her back to the foundation of her old house: If weak and stressed, it wobbles and eventually falls apart. If you have chronic back problems, I suggest jotting down what is occurring in your life at the time your back starts to act up. You may be very surprised at what your back is telling you.

Statistics cite that individuals who have low self-esteem or come from abused or turbulent backgrounds often have the most difficulty recovering from back problems.

Low self-esteem may simply translate into poor posture—slumping, rounded shoulders, and facing the world with your head down. These psychological situations may have to be dealt with at the same time you work through your backache.

REFLECTIVE PRACTICES TO SOOTHE AN ACHING BACK

I'm not going to tell you that the following practices will cure a backache. But they are preventive measures to help you and your backache in stressful situations. Remember, stress is one of the leading causes of back ailments. Many of these are practices that you would do well to incorporate into your daily life. Why? Because when people relax, slow down, and perceive what's going on in their body, they can begin to understand how breathing has a direct effect on stress, pain, and (surprise) a sore back. Here are eight suggestions for soothing an aching back:

1. Find a form or relaxation technique to practice daily. Maybe you need only to lie still for fifteen minutes, close your eyes, and relax your body. Focus on a point, quiet music, or the silence of your breath.

Meditation is another form of relaxation to ease stress. You don't need to have a guru to teach you to meditate, but some formal instruction may be helpful. There are several books and tapes to aid in relaxation. Check the appendix for suggestions.

A more active method of relaxation is sitting in your garden, quietly listening to the birds, or walking near the sea or in a park. Relaxation doesn't always translate into sitting stoically still in a lotus position. Quiet movement can also be a form of relaxation and meditation. Find what works for you and steal the time to practice it. Relaxation is the first step in breaking a stressful cycle.

2. Learn to pace your obligations. Don't bite off more than you can chew. If you relax for twenty minutes a day and cram the rest of the day with overbearing obligations, the benefits will be marginal.

3. Get enough rest.

4. Make sure you eat correctly and nourish your body.

5. Try to take as much control over your life as possible. This is especially important for anyone with chronic back pain.

6. Breathe! This one may sound silly, but how many times have you taken a deep breath before giving a speech, calling someone you admire for a date, or doing something that makes you nervous? When feeling stressful or anxious, stop, sit down, close your eyes, and take a few deep, gentle breaths.

7. If relaxing on your own proves too difficult, find a class that teaches relaxation techniques, or check with your doctor. Hospitals and HMOs all around the country offer classes with different techniques to relax and alleviate stress.

8. Communicate to friends, family, and coworkers your need for a few minutes to relax. If you've never meditated or taken fifteen minutes a day alone to be quiet, shutting a door and hanging a Don't Disturb sign can create uncomfortable feelings in a household or office.

Remember, prevention includes physical exercise. The following chapter offers exercises that you can either begin or finish your day with to keep your back in top condition.

Chapter 18

GROUND RULES: EXERCISES FOR THE BACK

Victor's career as a pilot abruptly came to a halt when his parachute didn't open. A drop from 3,500 feet broke several bones in his body. Lucky to be alive, Victor set about reconstructing his life and body. He left the hospital in a wheelchair. Determined, Victor did exercises and began working with a physical therapist. Today Victor trains the monkeys going into space for the French space program. Watching him, you see a tall, thin man, back erect, the picture of health. Few would know that Victor suffers from daily back pain and relies on swimming, yoga, and other exercise to manage it. Without incorporating exercises into his daily practice, the back pain would border on intolerable.

As with Victor, getting back in shape requires substantial backbone. There are several back exercise programs to choose from. Most incorporate a few of the same exercises. Some programs and books assure you that exercise is the answer to your back problem. This may be true in some cases, but it is not in others. You certainly won't know how exercise affects your back unless you try an exercise program. A word of warning, however: Exercises for your back should be incorporated into your life, not used only to heal a particular painful back episode. Ken is a classic example of what typically happens to the back-exercise candidate.

Ken, a researcher at a local university, woke up one morning and couldn't get out of bed. He stayed there hoping his back pain would subside. It didn't. A visit to his doctor, an X ray, and later a CAT scan confirmed a bulging disk. Pain medication, rest, and back school were prescribed. Ken remained in terrible pain for several weeks. Slowly, he eased off the pain medication and religiously began doing back exercises from his back school class. After a few months, his back felt fine. He changed his workstation so that he could work at the computer standing instead of sitting. This worked out well, and Ken began resuming normal activities. Unfortunately, the better he felt, the less he practiced his exercise program. A month later, while picking up his daughter, Ken had another back attack. Convinced that exercise at least prevented painful attacks, Ken resolved to stick with it.

In researching this book, I spoke to dozens of back sufferers who had been given exercises by specialists for their specific back problems. Most of the exercises required ten to fifteen minutes twice a day. None were excruciatingly difficult, and most of the people I spoke with began with great resolve. But 90 percent, although advised otherwise, quit doing exercises or curtailed the amount of time spent on exercises as soon as their backs felt better. And like Ken, most of them had a recurrence of back pain intense enough to force them to stay home from work or return to the doctor. If exercise decreases your pain, strengthens your muscles, or abates the pain of a back attack, you would do well to incorporate them into your daily life. At this juncture, the shape of your back rests primarily on your own shoulders.

NO QUICK FIX

Unless you were in a sudden serious accident, your back problem has evolved over time. Don't expect exercises for your back to work miracles overnight. An exercise program may take approximately six weeks before yielding any results. Six weeks of daily exercise, weekends included, is a good start. To give an exercise program a fair chance, allow a minimum of three months before determining conclusively how your back feels. Many back sufferers began an exercise program with the fervor of an avowed smoker ready to quit. Too often, the fervor lasts no more than two weeks, not long enough to help your back.

Do not begin an exercise program in the midst of an acute back attack. Wait until it subsides. Always have a physical therapist or trained expert show you how to do the exercises. The exercises should be carried out with the patience it requires to watch grass grow. Exercises are to help you promote suppleness and elasticity and to strengthen muscles; they are not aids to decrease pain during acute back pain.

BASIC BACK EXERCISES

These are good, solid exercises with or without a back problem. Do, however, check with your doctor before embarking on an exercise program if you have a specific back problem. Traditionally, the large muscles, such as the hamstrings and quadriceps, need strengthening with back pain. Remember, the muscles not only support the back but depend on each other to do their job.

When one set of muscles is weak, that muscular imbalance can create problems for your back.

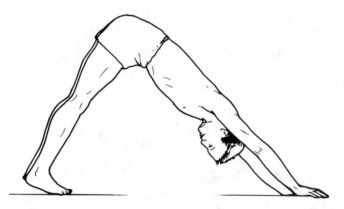

Illustration by Susan Spellman

Downward Facing Dog

Have you ever watched a dog stretch after a good sleep? Dogs stretch their spine, and the "downward facing dog" is a wonderful stretch for your back. Start on all fours with the palms of your hands and your knees on the floor, arms straight. Breathe out. Tuck your toes under and lift up your hips and buttocks, slowly. Straighten the legs as much as possible. Now stretch more, like a dog, so that your arms and legs are straight and your weight is back as far as you can make it on your heels. But be careful not to push your limits with the stretch. Stretch evenly and make a triangle with the floor. Bend your knees and sit gently down on your heels and relax.

Hold the "dog" for fifteen to thirty seconds and repeat twice.

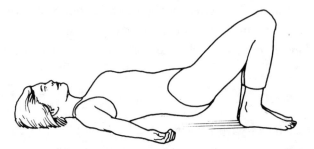

Illustration by Susan Spellman

The Classic Pelvic Tilt

Lie on the floor with your arms at your sides. Bend the knees, keeping your feet flat on the floor. Flatten the lower back against the floor. Tighten your stomach and buttocks muscles simultaneously. Hold this position for five seconds. Using your stomach muscles, slightly tilt the pelvis up and hold for five seconds. Relax the stomach muscles and feel the pelvis roll out of position. Repeat. The tilt strengthens the abdominal muscles that are so important for a healthy lower back.

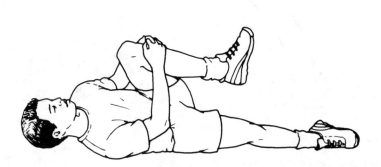

Illustration by Susan Spellman

Low Back Stretch

Lie flat on your back on the floor, hands at your sides. Bring one knee toward your chest, leaving the other leg extended. Hold the position for about five seconds, then release, returning to the original position. Alternate legs, keeping one stretched straight on the floor while bringing the opposite knee to the chest. Do not bring both knees to the chest at the same time; this puts strain on the disk.

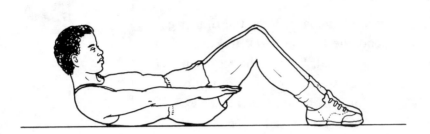

Illustration by Susan Spellman

The Abdominal Stretch or Sit-up

Lie on your back on the floor and bend your knees. Keep both feet flat on the floor. Reach with your arms toward your knees and slowly raise your head and shoulders off the floor ever so slightly. Make sure your low back is pressed flat against the floor, and hold for five seconds. Release and slowly let your head and arms roll back to the floor. Repeat. Do this exercise slowly, without jerking movements. Check with your doctor about the abdominal stretch if you have a precarious disk problem.

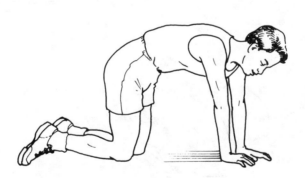

Illustration by Susan Spellman

The Cat

Okay, feline lovers, this is a wonderfully gentle exercise. Kneel on all fours like a cat. Your feet point backward; your hands face front. Exhale and push your back into a concave position, your head and tailbone pointed toward the ceiling. Hold for ten seconds. Inhale deeply while simultaneously moving the back into an arch, tightening the stomach and buttocks muscles. Now the chin and tailbone should point toward the floor. In this position, slowly exhale and stretch a little farther. Hold for ten seconds and return to the all-fours position. Repeat sequence five times.

Ankle Knee Pose

Stand facing a wall for support. Keep the right leg straight and bend the left leg back, taking the ankle with your left hand. Stretch the leg against the buttocks, using the right leg for support. Balance is important; this is not a beginner's exercise. If you've never stood balanced on one leg, this may be difficult. You want to keep your body erect, not bent or hunched over. The idea is to develop the quadriceps. Hold the position for five to ten seconds and switch legs.

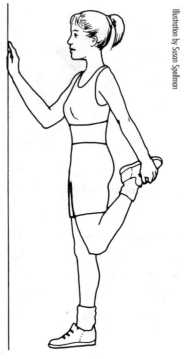

Illustration by Susan Spellman

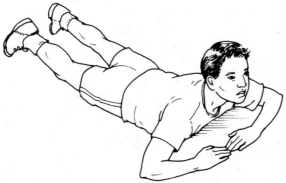

Illustration by Susan Spellman

The Cobra

Lie flat on your stomach, your forehead facedown. Place hands slightly beneath shoulders, fingers together, elbows extended out. Slowly, without pressure on the hands, raise the head a little, keeping legs together and weightless. Slowly raise the upper trunk by gently pushing hands against the floor ever so lightly. Very slowly the head should be tilted back, eyes looking upward, the spine curved throughout the movement. The head should be lifted slightly, keeping the curve in your upper back slight. Stay in this position for ten seconds. If your upper or lower back feels stressed, don't rise any farther; instead, lower a touch. You should not feel stress on the spine with the Cobra. It is the upper back, not the lower back, that should be working. Slowly lower this position in reverse order, your head touching the floor last. The Cobra is good for relieving tension throughout the back and spine. As your back becomes stronger, the head can rise higher, creating more of a curve in your upper back.

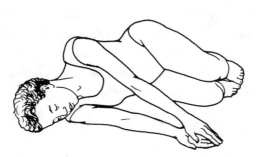

Illustration by Susan Spellman

Bedtime Stretch

This is very simple and has wonderful results. Begin by lying on your back with your knees bent. Make sure the upperback, shoulder blades, and midback are touching the floor. Gently roll to the right side, keeping both knees bent and together, and then extend the arms straight out in front of you. Slowly slide the left arm forward so that it moves across the right palm. Always keep your head in contact with the floor and the neck relaxed. Pause for a few seconds. Then, slide the left palm in the other direction so that it moves toward the inner arm. Pause for a few seconds and then return the palms together. Repeat five times, rest on your back, and practice on the left side. This stretch opens and stretches the upper back.

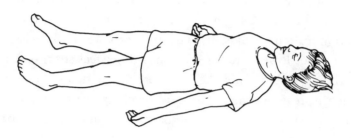

Illustration by Susan Spellman

Corpse or Relaxation Pose

Simply lie on your back on a mat or on the floor, hands to side and body relaxed. Tense your body, then release. Place legs slightly apart, roll the head from side-to-side, close your eyes and breathe. Bring the breath to the toes and relax the body all the way to the tip of the head. If you cannot do this in silence, because your active mind wanders, put on a classical music cassette or find a deep relaxation tape. Try this for fifteen minutes prior to going to bed. It relaxes the mind and the back.

Chapter 19

Easy-Does-It Remedies

How does it happen? One minute you are laughing, standing on your two feet; the next, you bend over to retrieve a piece of paper and you can't get up. Pain sears through your body like a bolt of lightning. The slightest movement is a challenge. You hobble over to the sofa and try to sit—too painful. You crawl onto the bed, bent in a fetal position, and wonder what to do. Should you take an aspirin and pray? Dial 911? Try to straighten your back? Contact the top orthopedist in your area? Tough out the pain?

So what should you do while you are down on your knees crippled and writhing in pain? The following are simple recommendations by a leading back specialist. They are not cures, but sensible suggestions to get you through the first painful forty-eight hours.

The Do's and Don'ts of a Back Attack

Do stay calm. I know, this may sound like a rather stupid recommendation to anyone who one minute is standing erect and the next minute is huddled into a jackknife position on the floor. If it's any comfort, statistics are in your favor. Remember, 80 percent of the back attacks heal without medical aid within a two-week period. The pain disappears on its own. Unfortunately, without understanding why your back went out or correcting bad back habits, you have the same percentage of a recurring back attack.

What if your back pain still doesn't go away, or intensifies? Do call your family doctor or internist and go in for a checkup.

TRAUMA AND THE BACK

Sandra was driving with her sister in a Volkswagen bug through Grand Junction, Colorado, when a policeman slowed the lane of traffic to a halt. Sandra twisted around in the passenger seat just in time to see a Mac truck smash the rear of the Volkswagen at 60 mph, thrusting Sandra forward. While an X ray found no obvious damage to Sandra's spine, the doctor recommended that Sandra see a physical therapist for her neck and back pain. Sandra returned to Chicago and for the next four years embarked on a search that nearly drove her out of her mind. Neither CAT scans nor MRIs showed spinal damage.

"My back ached constantly. Sometimes I was crippled up in pain and no one could find an obvious reason for the pain. I saw a neurologist, an orthopedist, and a physical therapist or two. I had massage and traction, used ice and heat, and visited a homeopath. I couldn't turn my neck and my life was literally falling apart. I had migraine headaches and decided to see a therapist after more than one doctor told me my pain was psychological." By chance or last resort, Sandra found a chiropractor in the phonebook. Diane Stevens was the first practitioner, recalls Sandra, that cured her pain. "She adjusted me, but she also believed in a mind, body, spirit connection. Diane Stevens insisted I combine nutrition, rest, and exercise with manipulation. The combination took me from pain to euphoria."

Unlike Sandra, Fran has not found a healer for her back pain. Fran's life changed in an instant when an uninsured motorist hit her car. Her car was a wreck, but at least her body felt fine . . . or so she thought. A few days later, Fran couldn't move. Her back spasmed, she canceled work. She visited a chiropractor, who suggested Fran get an MRI. The MRI showed nothing. Fran's pain intensified, and she had to take a leave of absence from her job as a social worker in a hospital. Fran tried ultrasound, physical therapy, and a painful epidural block.

- Do apply ice intermittently during the first 48 hours. Don't apply the ice directly to the skin, but make an ice wrap. This helps reduce swelling.

- Don't put heat on your back immediately. Heat tends to inflame the injured area. After two or three days, you can alternate heat and ice.

- Don't hobble around the first few days. Since movement is difficult, complete bed rest is called for, but only for a few days. Stay flat on your back if it provides pain relief.

- Don't stay in bed longer than a few days. Too many days in bed only slows down your recovery process.

- Do take aspirin, Tylenol, or ibuprofen. These act as anti-inflammatories. The combination of either aspirin, Tylenol, or ibuprofen and bed rest for a few days should get the healing process rolling.

- Do avoid painkillers. Painkillers and muscle relaxants do nothing for a sore back; they simply mask the pain.

- Do consult a doctor if you have shooting pain in your buttocks or leg or numbness in your leg. This may indicate a serious disk injury.

- Don't rush into surgery for a disk injury. Surgery is an option, but not necessarily a given. Be aware of the doctor who puts you on the surgery schedule without trying a conservative approach first.

- Do go immediately to your doctor's office or the emergency room if you have a sudden loss of bowel, bladder, or neurological control. This is a red flag, and if not treated immediately, it can result in severe and permanent nerve damage.

- Don't try to drive if you're hunched over in pain.

- Don't try to lift anything, even your toddler.

- Don't work at your desk on that overdue report.

- Do try to stretch sore muscles gently after pain has eased.

"The epidural was the low point in this ordeal. It didn't work, and when the doctor suggested I try another one, I walked out of his office," Fran recalls.

Her mother sent her John Sarno's books on pain relief. Fran recognized her pain was not in her mind. To add pain to injury, a small area of her back caved in. Fran is 5'1" and weighs 100 pounds. The hole looked like a crater.

"No one had a clue to what was wrong with my back. But one thing was quite obvious to the naked eye—a portion of my back had collapsed," said Fran.

After several months off work, a bout with painkillers, and too much time in bed, Fran's physical therapist worked with Fran's back muscles to rectify the hole. It did not resolve the pain. It took a small electrical TENS machine to ease Fran's pain. By stimulating the muscles, Fran was able to control the pain. Fran went back to work and to this day carries the TENS machine with her wherever she goes. Her pain, although diminished, sometimes acutely returns.

An acute back attack strikes with a vengeance, often without indication, and it takes your breath away. The unrelenting pain is usually centered in the lower back. A nasty surprise, it drives you to your knees on the ninth hole of your best golf game ever; prevents you from retrieving your two-year-old from the infant car seat; and dumbfounds someone who has never experienced a back episode. Although 80 percent of these back attacks subside within ten days or two weeks, the moment is agonizing.

Speculation shrouds a sudden back revolt. Many times a back attack starts with stress and works its way into a painful spasm. Often we ignore the stress, thus ignoring even the most predominant signals. Susan is a good example of not acknowledging her back trouble. Scheduled to start a new job, life became hectic around the departure from her old job. A person who doesn't like to leave anything undone, Susan worked relentlessly until her last day. The day before starting her new position, she threw her back out. A stoic, and not wanting to make a bad showing at the beginning of a new job, she mustered the strength and somehow managed to start her new position as scheduled. But with each passing hour, the pain intensified. By three o'clock she could not move. Her back spasm had turned into a full-blown, excruciatingly painful back attack. She called her husband, who suggested a doctor. Susan opted for home remedies.

Remedies

There are some basic remedies and suggestions that specialists concur might support a painful situation in an emergency.

If you are alone, try and get help. This may mean crawling to the nearest telephone and dialing a spouse or a friend. Let someone who is nearby gently help you. At this juncture the choice is clearly up to you: Call your doctor or chiropractor, or go home and recline in bed.

If seeing a physician is your chosen route, you will most likely be given a prescription for pain medication and sent home with instructions to lie flat on your back and stay quiet and rest.

If you do not go to a practitioner and choose to self-medicate, your best choice of nonprescribed drugs should include a couple of aspirins or ibuprofen. If medication, whether prescribed or nonprescribed, is the route you choose to take, do so immediately. Do not, however, overmedicate yourself.

Bed Rest?

With an acute back attack you will not be able to do anything but lie still. Any movement, no matter how slight, causes excruciating pain. Back experts agree that a few days in bed should get you back on your feet—maybe not up and about like before, but moving. If after two or three days in bed the pain has not diminished, call your doctor.

At one time doctors advised extensive bed rest. Today, however, research indicates that prolonged bed rest is more of a hindrance than a help to your ailing back. But while you are in bed, your rest should be absolute: lying perfectly still on your back, getting up only to use the bathroom.

Absolute bed rest for an active person can be a challenge. Lying around ruminating about the pain in your back can be a bore. Read a book or watch TV, but *do not move about*. The tendency to get back in motion the moment the pain dissipates is tempting. For a few days, anyway, give your back the well-deserved rest it needs.

Supine Positions

According to Edward A. Abraham's book *Freedom from Back Pain,* lying flat on your back is the best position when you're experiencing a painful back episode. Putting a pillow under the knees is helpful. This takes the pressure off the sciatic nerve—the one that feels like a lightning bolt if you move. The fetal position, where you lie on your side and draw your knees up toward your chest, may also feel comfortable. Listen to your body; it will tell you which position is best for your back. If a supine position is painful, turn over onto your stomach.

Hot or Cold

Both heat and cold are effective in alleviating some of the pain that results from muscle or ligament strain. Heat increases the blood flow or circulation to the deep tissues, and ice works to deaden the nerve perception and prevent swelling. Some people prefer heat, others prefer ice. Alternating the two may bring relief. Do not apply a chunk of ice or a heating pad directly to the skin. And do not overchill or overheat the area. Ten to fifteen minutes each should be the maximum for either therapy.

Massage

I know, the thought of having someone touch your back during an acute back attack is enough to make you cringe. But after the initial pain has subsided, a massage may help the muscles to relax. Repeated gentle stroking brings circulation to the area, which in turn relaxes and warms.

Generally, two types of massage are practiced: the Swedish, a light stroking in one direction with deep pressure in another, and shiatsu, based on the concept of energy pathways or meridians. Shiatsu, more concerned with organs than with muscles, holds that a block in an organ, such as a kidney, can affect your back. Regardless of the method you choose, touch is a wonderful stimulus for relaxation and alleviating tension.

After the Initial Attack, Then What?

While your back may take a few weeks to a few months to feel as if it belongs to you again, you must make an effort to perform basic activities. Walking, stretching, and moving about are guaranteed to speed up the recovery process and get your back into shape. Remember, your back will not heal without your help. Like steering a car in the right direction, you have to commandeer your back's recuperation. You wouldn't push a new car to its maximum limit the first few weeks you owned it, nor should you do the same to your back. Don't stress your back, but do make an effort to move. Inactivity only weakens the back muscles.

OTHER TREATMENT MODALITIES ALONG THE ROAD TO RECUPERATION

Your doctor or chiropractor may suggest some electronic treatments along the way. These modalities are generally used in the initial phases of treatment to ease discomfort.

Diathermy and Ultrasound

Both of these treatments stimulate tissue under the skin by generating heat, which in turn calms the nerves and muscles that are causing pain. The treatment, performed in a medical office or clinic, works by focusing ultrasound or a mild electrical charge (diathermy) on the affected area. While the results may occur quickly, they are usually only temporary.

TENS (Transcutaneous Electrical Nerve Stimulation)

TENS uses electrodes connected to an electrical signal generator to bring about nerve impulses with a sporadic pulsing sensation. It acts to reduce pain. The portable mechanism is about the size of a small pocket radio with wires attached. You attach it to your waist. The electrodes at the end of the wires are placed near the spine. Here a light current is emitted to block the pain.

You can purchase or rent a TENS unit. Usage should be temporary, and studies show relief is, again, only temporary. Although many who try TENS find only temporary relief, for someone like Fran, TENS allowed her to continue her normal life.

Biofeedback

In biofeedback, sophisticated electronic equipment connects the individual to a machine that monitors muscle tension. The machine feeds back the level of existing tension by emitting a series of electronic beeps. When the muscles become tense, the sounds increase in both volume and frequency. When the muscles are relaxed, the volume and frequency both decrease. The technique induces deep muscle relaxation. With practice, the individual learns to relax tense muscles consciously. As the individual slows down the auditory signals, muscle tension is reduced. Biofeedback is part of many pain clinics.

Other Orthopedic Paraphernalia

A variety of braces, corsets, and other appliances give support to your back. A few times when my back moved out of place and I needed to sit at the computer, I put a corset on to support my spine while working and then removed it afterward. Something tight around the abdomen and lower spine may offer temporary relief. Any form of corset, however, should be temporary.

In the throes of a back attack, exercise sounds as probable as a voyage to the moon. Chances are, though, you're a healthy statistic, and your back pain will dissipate in a few weeks. You'll be up and ready to jump back into the game, your back pain long forgotten. Read chapter 20 prior to returning to the playing field. You may have to modify your technique and possibly change your game plan.

Chapter 20

SPORTS AND YOUR BACK

A competitive sports enthusiast and dancer, I certainly felt that years on tennis courts, mountains, and the dance floor protected my body from aging. Yet in my third decade of life, my joints began making funny noises, and my back revolted while doing barre warm-ups in a ballet class.

Perplexed and in severe pain, I had little choice but to hobble to a doctor. I went to a wise old chiropractor whose advice confirmed my athletic suspicion: Find a more gentle form of exercise; your body is telling you something. His advice, which I was in no position not to take, relegated this once graceful dancer to walking, swimming, and yoga. I resisted at first, but in time I began to see his reasoning. What I neglected to understand until researching this book was while all those years on the dance floor, tennis court, and mountains had kept me fit, with a nice trim body, my tendency to play hard had indeed been unkind to my back.

Sports are a wonderful way to stay in shape. Anyone concerned with his or her health understands how vital activity is for the body and mind. Every current publication on the back discusses the merits of exercise in maintaining a healthy spine. For anyone who has spent years avidly exercising, the knowledge that continuous exercise demands a degree of commitment is well understood.

You know yourself better than anyone else: How persistent are you? Will you persist with exercise once a back attack has subsided, or make exercise an integral part of your lifestyle?

Many first-time back sufferers begin a master plan of continuing exercise. They start with wonderful intentions. But as pain diminishes or disappears, out the window go the good intentions. Excuses are pertinent. There's difficulty in maintaining a time-consuming program, or time constraints don't allow a drive across town to the nearest gym or pool. If you cannot or do not have the inclination to maintain a resolute exercise program for your back, then choose a sport that you enjoy, and maintain it.

Many of the following sports are not designed specifically to simply strengthen the back. But stretching and warming up prior to your sport of choice should always precede a vigorous exercise session, thus strengthening your back.

To appreciate the role of exercise in back prevention, you must understand that back ailments commonly fall under strains, sprains, and arthritic pain. Weak muscles and ligaments spell trouble for your back. The interdependent strength of the spine is created through the muscle, ligament, and connective tissue working cohesively together. Exercise strengthens all these elements.

Arthritic conditions and aging may not be reversed, but throughout your life the spine strives to repair and compensate for much of the degenerative changes that occur. Remember, though, that while aging is inevitable, and many conditions such as arthritis are part of the aging process, being in poor condition is completely avoidable—and reversible.

So with all this in mind, what is the best sport for your back? Depending on the type of back condition you have, you may first want to check with your physician or sports doctor before proceeding with a vigorous sport. Many sports score high on the list of good choices, while others score low. Obviously, if you are involved in a sport or exercise similar to my ballet experience and you keep experiencing pain or injury, it is time to move on to something less brutal. Find the exercise or sport that works for you. Above all, remember the importance of stretching and limbering up before proceeding with any sport.

What the Experts Say

Ballet

The human body was not designed to withstand the strain of ballet's many convoluted positions. Sorry, ballet fanatics. Ballet, with all its grace and elegance, is a high risk for your back. The demanding training and arching of the back ultimately creates problems. Facet and hip-joint pain from hyperextension and rotary movements are also detrimental to a healthy back.

Bowling

Bowling can be risky if you already suffer with a bad back. Your leg is in a flexed position, and the weight of the ball is on one side of the body only. This posture can strain both the disks of the lumbar spine and opposite hip joint. Avoid using a heavier ball than is necessary. If you have chronic back pain, try wearing a corset while bowling.

Bicycling

Bicycling is an overall good aerobic conditioner, but it has limited advantages to strengthening the back muscles. In many cases, if seats, handlebars, and frames aren't properly adjusted, back pain may be increased. Your best bet is not to jump on your friend's bike and pedal off into the sunset. If you don't have a bike of your own, adjust the bicycle to your needs. Always set the bike accurately for your needs, whether pedaling outside or inside on an exercise bike. Don't purchase a bike that requires you to be stretched over to reach the handlebars. Maintain good posture while bicycling. And check out the following:

Frame. Try several bicycles and find the frame that fits your height and weight.

Seat. Seats are adjustable and should give you a good leg extension when pedaling.

Handlebars. Some newer bikes come with higher handlebars, which allow for a more upright position when bicycling.

Pedals. While you are sitting on the bike, your leg should be fully extended, but you should not lock your knees when pedaling.

The newer mountain bike is better for your back than the older, 10-speed bicycles, where you had to lean forward. Weight may also be a factor for you if you have to lift a bicycle. The newer, more expensive bikes can be extremely lightweight. Remember, if you have to lift a bicycle on and off a rack, lift with your knees, not your back.

Bodybuilding

For decades bodybuilding belonged to the men. Now, it's a co-ed sport that if done correctly tones and beautifies the body. Is weightlifting good for your back, though? Some doctors place weightlifting on the nix list, to be approached with caution if you are prone to back problems.

If you do not have back problems, moderation is advised. Build your resistance slowly. The greatest risk in bodybuilding is with heavy weights. Lifting more than you can handle can potentially create stress fracture, muscle strain, and ligament problems. If bodybuilding is your favorite sport, choose lighter weights and strive for repetition.

Consider your age when lifting, as well as the age of your spine. The Texas Back Institute recommends lifting belts for its patients in labor-intensive jobs. A lifting belt supports the back, and although the merits of a lifting belt are controversial, it may help prevent a back injury.

There is good news about weight-bearing exercise for women. A recent study showed that weight-bearing exercise helps ameliorate the osteoporatic process, even in older women. Stay away from rowing machines if you have a bad back, though. It's too much of a load on the spine.

Diving

Diving is not recommended for a chronic back pain sufferer. Any dive that demands hyperextension, like the jackknife, stresses the lower back. Needless to say, diving in shallow water can cause severe neck or spinal injuries. Always check the depth of the water before diving.

Golf

Many enjoy golf throughout their entire life. It is a low-impact sport, a relaxing way to spend the weekend. But it is also considered one of those borderline sports—it may never affect your back, but if it does, watch out. The trouble in golf is with the follow-through swing of the club. As you swing, the trunk of the body is often poorly controlled. If you already have a back injury, this leaves you vulnerable to more problems.

Gymnastics

Gymnastics is a high-risk sport with or without back problems. The wear and tear to the facet joints from severe hyperextension of the spine creates problems later in life. Again, the human body is not designed to extend to the degree it must for several gymnastic postures. If your child is interested in gymnastics, make sure the instructor is well trained, understands the importance of good spotting, and does not push a child to the point of exhaustion.

Walking

Walking is good for everything—your heart, soul, and back. Invest in a pair of good walking shoes, and stay on flat land if hills give your back problems. Walk with intention, not with your hands shoved in your pockets and your head down. Concentrate on keeping your abdominals tucked in when walking.

Jogging

Jogging is probably enjoyed by more people than any other sport at this time. Whether you're a marathon runner or just out for a few laps around the block, jogging is good for the heart and legs, though the jarring sometimes affects joints and disks. To lessen the impact, invest in good running shoes. Run on grass or dirt, not cement. With back problems, shorter runs are better than long, marathon-type stints.

Martial Arts

Martial arts are not considered a high risk for back sufferers. This may be due to the centering of the body and a clear understanding of the body and mind working together. Many who suffer from mild back pain participate in martial arts. The warm-up in martial arts is as important as the martial art itself.

Swimming

Swimming provides excellent shoulder and upper-body strengthening. There is no jarring or bouncing of the spine with this sport. During pregnancy, swimming can make the body feel almost weightless and is a good way to stay in condition. Swimming, however, is not an exercise that strengthens the spine as much as it does the upper body, legs, and arms. The breaststroke is not your best bet if you have a back problem. The crawl should be done in a succinct, gentle rhythm without stressing the back or neck. The sidestroke and backstroke are your safest bet if you are in dire back pain.

Tennis

People with back problems often continue to play tennis. Many back problems in tennis stem from the high degree of body rotation and extension required to play an aggressive game of tennis. Tennis, however, does not have to be played as aggressively as you once might have attacked it. One of the most difficult moves for a tennis player to acquire after a back injury is to not feel a compelling need to go after some of the most difficult and strenuous shots on the court.

Posture is of prime importance in tennis, and it surely is paramount to both a good tennis game and a functioning back. A good tennis stance, with knees bent and abdominal muscles tightened, helps the back. Hit the ball at shoulder height, and use the hips and knees rather than the lumbar spine when hitting knee-high returns. Be careful with your lumbar extension when serving. If a serious back injury prevents you from playing the tennis game you once conquered, begin slowly by hitting tennis balls against a backboard. This allows you to better regain good posture and control your body movements.

Skiing

Skiing has its own set of risks, especially when performed by the weekend warrior or once-a-year enthusiast. Many people who either water-ski or downhill ski do so without being in good physical condition. Waterskiing can be strenuous on the back, and downhill skiing adds risk with twisting the spine and crashing in oddball positions, not to mention the array of paraphernalia one has to haul just to get onto the mountain. So does this mean just because you don't live on the Great Lakes or in the Rocky Mountains you should stay away? No; what it means for your back is that if you want to avoid risk, get into shape with a conditioning program at least a month or two before your outing. An avid mountain skier, raised in a Southern California town,

I spent many hours with my back against a wall, knees bent, as if sitting on a chair. Lowering my body until my thighs were parallel with the floor, I sat for small, increasing increments of time, building up leg muscles for the slopes.

The greatest risk for your back—or other limbs for that matter—while snow skiing is falling wrong. Find slopes that don't challenge your back. In waterskiing, maintain a good speed and let go when you fall or when your back begins to ache. Cross-country skiing, by the way, is excellent exercise for both your heart and your back.

Team Sports

Obviously, team sports are a bit more tricky when it comes to your back. You don't have as much control with all the turning, twisting, or being jostled about. Sports such as soccer, football, rugby, and hockey carry a much greater risk for anyone with a back problem.

Contact sports entail kicking, twisting, sudden body movements, and high speed. Combine this with running or skating at the same time, and you can see why these sports could cause your back a great many problems. You may participate in a team sport and, with a good warm up and caution, never have an injury. But if you already have a back problem, you might consider a gentler individual sport.

Equipment

Whatever your choice of sport, make sure you use good equipment. It doesn't have to be the top brand name on the market, but it should be good. Experiment with various types before settling on a particular racket or bicycle, for example. Sports equipment has altered drastically in the last decade. Just because it's new and in vogue this year may not mean that it's best for your back problem now or ten years from now.

So now that you're in shape, have great body mechanics, and mindfully acknowledge your spine in stressful times, what else could possibly go wrong with your back? Getting up and going to work!

Chapter 21

TRAVELING WITH BACK PAIN

Cori travels extensively for work. She's in good physical shape, and she exercises and practices yoga. Cori has a job that many people envy: playing and writing about golf. Cori also travels a lot. So, she was surprised when on a recent flight from California to Honolulu she arrived in Honolulu cringing with back pain. "The flight was crowded and I was seated in the last row, the one that didn't recline. It was a terrible flight, stressful and uncomfortable, and apparently too much for my back. I certainly wasn't in any condition to play golf when I arrived," recalls Cori.

Cori couldn't go to bed with ice packs, or stretch out on the beach; she had a golf tournament the next day. The concierge at her hotel gave her the name of a massage therapist who Cori swears saved her golf game. "I've never played better. The masseuse kneaded and pummeled the spasm with some kind of New Age Hawaiian technique. Bliss replaced pain and I was able to relax enough to play golf. Now, if I have a big tournament, I try and schedule a massage or two in advance. I know it sounds decadent, and yes, it's expensive, but it works," she claims.

Traveling with a bad back is a liability—you never know when its going to act up. Back flair-ups never discriminate geographically or economically—they can bother you on a bus in Katmandu or aboard a luxury liner in the Caribbean. It doesn't matter if you've booked yourself into a five-star chateau or you are camping, a back attack puts a crimp in your vacation plans. There are two options for your back while on the road: preventive measures or cultivate extraordinary survival skills.

AIR TRAVEL

Many individuals who don't typically suffer from chronic back pain find that long flights trigger either neck or back spasms. And if airline service continues to decline in coach class, it's likely that more people will walk off planes grumbling about the pain piercing their backs. Cori did not stop flying, nor will you or I. But, like Cori, who now carries an inflatable neck pillow and a plastic collapsible footstool to accommodate her back, there are a handful of solutions.

Choosing a Seat

Boarding airlines is no longer what it used to be. If you fly economy, you may not even be able to choose a seat until you arrive at the airport. Avoid this if possible. Ask what type of plane you will fly on and what the seating arrangements are like. Lack of leg room and sardinelike cell space are the two biggest complaints from irate frequent flyers. Factor in less available nonstop flights and it may take you more time than it took the Wright Brothers to cross the Atlantic to arrive at your destination. None of this bodes well for a bad back. Your back can suffer during flights, sometimes for several days afterward.

If you can upgrade or afford to fly business class, it's a better scenario for your back and your psyche. It's the difference between riding in a Rolls Royce and a Volkswagen. The seats are wider, cushier, more comfortable. Leg room is more extensive, leg rests rise, and seats recline. There is also space to move your bones about, and the atmosphere is generally less hectic. That said, most of us don't fly first or business class, so we have to learn to be creative.

Creatively start by packing a little extra back paraphernalia. Speaking of bags, check them in. Avoid toting luggage on your shoulder through the airport or hoisting heavy bags in the overhead compartment if you suffer from back pain. Instead, pack a neck pillow and a small back pillow and try to avoid the middle seat. Aisle seats allow you the freedom to get up, move around, and stretch your legs. If an aisle seat isn't available, ask for a window seat, which gives you something to lean on, so your head isn't bobbing around, creating all sorts of problems for your neck when you snooze during a flight.

If you are scheduled to fly and your back is in pain, wear a corset, which can be purchased in any back store or from a chiropractor. A corset braces both your abdominal muscles and lower back and will prevent you from slumping in your seat. If you suspect your back will act up aboard a flight, carry a package of frozen peas or frozen corn to place behind your lower back. Tennis balls have the same effect; they deflect the spasm, keeping you sitting upright. Watch your reading position. Make sure your head isn't jutting forward and your shoulders aren't hunched over a book. People read on long flights and work on computers. Try to be as ergonomic as possible while in the air. Speaking of air, practice a few breathing techniques; they relax not only your mind, but your entire body. If you are too inhibited to practice relaxation breathing, carry a relaxation cassette and plug it in.

Airport Etiquette

I've seen people squatting in airports, stretching against walls, and lying on the floor in airports, all to relieve back pain. Once in Seattle, I noticed a well-dressed man stretched on his stomach near the baggage claim. He slowly moved into a cobra posture while he waited for his baggage. If you have a long flight and a lay-over between flights, walk around the airport. When you arrive at your destination, hail a porter to retrieve and carry your luggage, and tip him well.

ACCOMMODATIONS

Unless you're staying in a youth hostel, or traveling on $25 a day, you probably have mattress options. Request a hard, firm mattress for sleeping. Take a hot shower and relax your muscles before sightseeing or conferences. If your hotel has a jacuzzi or spa, indulge, indulge, indulge. Many hotels have masseuses or spas. Get a massage, but make sure the person pummeling you knows that you have a bad back.

TRAIN TRAVEL

The benefit of train travel is that you can get up and walk around. It's too slow for those who are in a hurry to get to a destination, but it can be relaxing. If you travel by train in Europe, you have first and second class options as you do in many parts of Asia. Typically, second class trains in Europe are splendid, and Japan and many European countries also have bullet trains to speed you to your destination. Carry a pillow or towel to roll behind your lower back if you are in pain.

The biggest problem with train travel is that you may have to carry your own luggage on and off the platform. Pack lightly because heaving large bags up the steps of a train car and off again is not a harmonious solution for a sensitive back.

CAR

When traveling by car, stop and get out as much as possible to walk or stretch. Purchase either a back or seat cushion designed especially for driving.

EMERGENCIES ON THE ROAD AND IN DISTANT LANDS

We all know people who have broken limbs while traveling, but the story that sticks with me is about a man who went to Bali, fell from a ledge, and broke his back. Fortunately, he made it home and wrote about the incident. It's much more likely that you'll catch a cold than you will break your back anywhere, but back spasms often occur on the road. Do abroad what you would do at home. Unless it's an emergency, avoid rushing to the hospital. If you take muscle relaxants at home for back pain, carry a few with you. Do not push yourself to sightsee with a bad back. And, bring good walking shoes no matter where you travel.

Chapter 22

ERGONOMICS AND YOUR BACK

Ergonomics, the study of equipment design, came into being in order to reduce operator fatigue and discomfort. But it's not just for the workplace; it should be a component of your everyday life if you suffer with back problems. The advent of working on the computer completely changed the work modality; arduous hours of repetitive motion has also given rise to repetitive-type injury and lawsuits. Because the workplace has changed so drastically in the last few decades, most business personnel recognize that a comfortable workstation must accommodate more than one position over the period of a day. All too often one overlooks the requirements of a good work space. Suddenly your back aches, your neck is tight, and your body feels tense and tired. We grumble that it's just too expensive to buy the right chair or change our desk. I, too, was one of those grumblers.

I had spent what seemed to me a small fortune on a computer. I went hog-wild—top-of-the-line software, a color monitor. I plunked my new machine atop my old-fashioned, but roomy teacher's desk, pulled up a kitchen chair, and began writing. Within a few months my neck revolted, my back muscles were sore, and I began having pain across my sternum. My husband suggested I buy a good chair.

No way. I wasn't about to buy an expensive chair simply to sit in. I would, however, consider parting with my desk, which had been designed for correcting papers, not for computer work. But my screen was too high; I had to look up at it. Maybe a change in height would correct my aching neck and back.

I went shopping and found a computer table. Now the keyboard and monitor were the perfect height, but I still had backaches. My husband kept harping about my chair.

"Okay," I said. "I'll go to an ergonomic shop, but don't expect me to plunk down several hundred dollars for a chair."

Of course, once I started shopping, my backside and my back could detect the difference in chairs. Then the saleswoman said that she noticed an interesting phenomenon with her clientele. Individuals spent a lot of money on computer equipment but neglected to enhance the most important aspect of their work space, their seat and their desk. You guessed it. I walked out of her shop with an expensive chair—not top-of-the-line, but adequate for my needs—and believe me, the purchase of that ergonomically designed chair has served my backside, back, arms, and posture well. I hate to admit it, but my husband was right.

ERGONOMIC SCHOOLS OF THOUGHT

Ergonomics is a relatively new field, yet there are different schools of thought. Eileen Vollowitz, P.T, founder of Back Designs in Berkeley, California, explains that active and passive approaches are a contentious question among experts. Should you use an arm rest or no arm rest, a tiny back chair or a big back chair? Should you sit or stand? All this depends on your lifestyle and the expert recommending what type of chair you should be sitting in.

A passive approach means that you are completely supported while you sit. You're relaxed; the chair can recline; and your neck, back, and arms are supported by the chair. The active approach recommends a saddlelike seat which you straddle. These seats stimulate all postural muscles as though you were standing. Bodywork practitioners tend to be inclined toward a more active approach; while the passive approach has traditionally been more clinically supported. Your job may dictate whether you sit in an active or passive seat. If your job requires you to manipulate things and move around, the straddle seat might be a good option. But if your job is tied to hours of conferences or desk work, you may choose a passive-style chair.

As another component of your workspace, keyboards can also be passive or active. The newest approach to keyboarding is the float technique. You move your hands, wrists, and head as you would if you were playing a piano; the wrists do not remain static. A passive chair is not the best option with this method because you sit as you would at a piano—erect and squarely on a seat with a twelve-inch back. Many of the newer ergonomic keyboards have passive designs and include wrist rests which must be removed to use the keyboard actively.

Look for more changes in the ergonomic field, but it may be best to obtain a few expert opinions if you're not sure which approach works best for you. Try both and see what feels best. Again, passive or active may depend on your job and particular back or neck problem.

The Ideal Workstation for Computer Use

A screen angled improperly creates postural problems. Posture always follows the eyes. A low screen forces your head forward and down. This strains the neck and back. If your screen is too low, place it on top of the computer unit or a stack of books.

If your computer screen is too high, it may cause your head to tilt back and your chin to protrude forward. This causes neck strain. One solution is to move the screen off the computer unit. If your screen is too far away, your head thrusts forward and you may slump and strain both the back and neck. Move closer to the screen. How close is too close? Keep the computer screen an arm's distance away from you. The distance from your screen to your eyes should be about the same distance you maintain between your eyes and usual reading material.

The Chair

Your seat contours should follow the contours of your back. Get a chair that supports your back and has armrests. Ideally, your chair should have a control to move the seat up and down, forward and backward. You should also be able to angle your thighs.

Consider these questions when purchasing a chair: Does your backrest recline and support your low back and upper back, and furthermore does it have a height adjustment? Chairs without backrest height adjustment fit few people. Are there adjustment controls, and are they easy to reach? Are armrests slightly higher than the point of your bent elbow? (They should be.) Does your chair swivel, allowing you to adjust your reach and line of vision without twisting your body? Does your seat support your thighs while your feet or legs rest comfortably on the floor, and is it at least two inches wider than you are?

The Keyboard

Arms should be relaxed at your side, with elbows a few inches from your body. Minimize your reach. If you adjust your chair, be sure to readjust the keyboard.

The Desk

Desk height is important in relationship to your keyboard. If you do not work at a computer table and your surface is nonadjustable, try some alternatives. If your desk is too high, try raising your chair and putting a stool beneath your feet. If your desk is too low, add blocks to the table legs to elevate the desk. Most work surfaces are a standard twenty-eight to thirty inches, which is a good height for people between 5'8" to 5'10". If you are taller or shorter, you may need to vary the height to fit you.

The Copy Stand

If documents are part of your workday, get a stand on which to mount the papers. Put your documents in the same place and at the same height as the screen. You can mount a stand on your screen or buy a portable one. Looking down at documents causes tremendous neck and upper back strain.

The Ergonomic Stretch

This is a simple exercise that can be done in your office or when you take a computer break. It is marvelous for upper and lower back stress that occurs while working at a desk or computer. Stand with your feet shoulder width apart, elbows bent, and palms together. Reach hands toward the sky without arching your lower back, while keeping the elbows as close as you can get them. Spread the arms into a "V" position, palms facing in, but do not lift your shoulders. Then drop your arms, bending the elbows into an "L" position. Slowly bring the arms behind your back, and then cross the palms, if possible. Repeat this exercise between five and ten times.

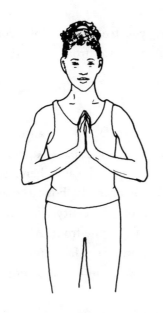

Illustration by Susan Spellman

STAND

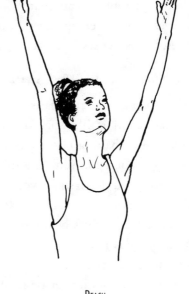

REACH

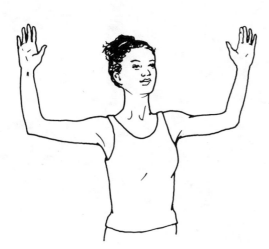

DROP

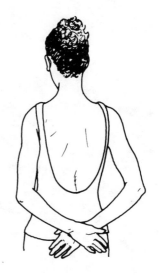

SLOWLY

Movement

Keep moving; motion and change of position make you feel better. Take computer breaks every hour. Get up, stretch, move about, but get away from the screen. Give your eyes, hands, wrists, and back a break.

I Can't Afford a New Work Station

You may not need to purchase a new computer setup. In fact, you can often work around an uncomfortable work situation. You may need to add a back support pillow in lieu of a new chair, or else a versatile support that you can take anywhere. You may need a consultation and someone to show you how to sit properly, how to place your papers so that you don't strain your eyes or neck. Look for a specialty store that offers consultation, advice, books, and a catalogue of products to choose from. Always ask for cost-effective alternatives before making an expensive purchase. Make sure the person you speak with is not just a salesperson, but someone who understands ergonomics and your particular problem.

Ergonomics can no longer be ignored, particularly with changes in the workplace. See the appendix for stores that serve the back, the workplace, and the future.

FINAL WORDS

Richard A. Deyo, professor in the departments of medicine and health services at the University of Washington writes, "Consider the following paradox, the American economy is increasingly post-industrial, with less heavy labor, more automation, and more robotics; and medicine has consistently improved diagnostic imaging of the spine and developed new forms of surgical and non0surgical therapy. But work disability caused by back pain has steadily risen." While the Information Superhighway has simplified our lives in numerous ways, it has also been unkind to the spine and filled our daily lives with more stress than many of us ever imagined. Whether we work from our desks at home, in an office, or on the road, we all sit much more than we should, spending long hours in front of a screen, in airports, in cars, and less time outdoors moving about.

More people than ever before suffer from back pain. Can we alter this epidemic? Yes, but not with the sedentary lifestyle that Western culture has embraced. A healthy back in the next century deems moving back to basics—walking, getting outside more, and keeping our bodies and minds fit. Whatever we can do to lower or eliminate stress helps the backbone. This might require saying no to more hours at the computer or in front of your favorite television program. It will most definitely require some ingenuity and creativity, but in the end, I believe it is worth it—just ask anyone who suffers with a bad back.

Medical science will continue its heroic endeavor to unravel the mysteries surrounding back pain. Diagnostic testing will continue to improve, and spine surgery will become less of an ordeal. Alternative healing and nurturing the human spirit will find their way into traditional modalities. With a little care and courage, we are entrusted as both guardian and keeper of that precious anatomical structure, the spine.

APPENDIX

Chapter 2

SPINA BIFIDA ASSOCIATION OF AMERICA
4590 MacArthur Blvd., N.W., Suite 250
Washington, DC 20007-4226
1-800-621-3141
For a staff member: (202) 944-3285
Fax: (202) 944-3295

PARENT INFORMATION CENTER
P.O. Box 2405
Concord, NH 03302-2405
(603) 224-7005
Fax: (603) 224-4365
E-mail: picnh@aol.com
Provides information and support.

EXCEPTIONAL PARENT MAGAZINE
555 Kinderkamack Road
Oradell, NJ 07649
1-800-372-7368
(201) 634-6550
Fax: (201) 634-6599
Web site: www.pedianet.com

Chapter 3

THE ARTHRITIS & BACK PAIN CENTER
The Swezey Institute Building
1328 16th Street
Santa Monica, CA 90404
(310) 394-1113

ARTHRITIS FOUNDATION
P.O. Box 19000
Atlanta, GA 30326
1-800-283-7800

FIBROMYALGIA NETWORK
P.O. Box 31750
Tucson, AZ 85751
(520) 290-5508
Web site: www.fmnetnews.com

NATIONAL INSTITUTE OF NEUROLOGICAL
    DISORDERS AND STROKES
P.O. Box 5801
Bldg. 31, Rm. 8A-06 MSC-2540
31 Center Drive
Bethesda, MD 20892-2540
1-800-352-9424
Offers free publications and pamphlets on
back pain.

ANKYLOSING SPONDYLITIS ASSOCIATION
511 N. La Cienega, Suite 216
Los Angeles, CA 90048
(310) 652-0609

Chapter 4

NATIONAL OSTEOPOROSIS FOUNDATION
1150 17th Street, N.W., Suite 500
Washington, DC 20036-4603
(202) 223-2226
1-800-223-9994
Web site: www.nof.org

SCOLIOSIS RESEARCH SOCIETY
6300 North River Road, Suite 727
Rosemont, IL 60018-4226
(847) 698-1627
Web site: www.srs.org

SCOLIOSIS ASSOCIATION, INC.
P.O. Box 811705
Boca Raton, FL 33481-1705
1-800-800-0669

Chapter 5

AMERICAN PAIN SOCIETY
4700 West Lake Avenue
Glenview, IL 60025-1485
(847) 375-4715
Web site: www.ampainsoc.org
A professional organization of physicians
and pain-management experts. Provides
referrals.

INTERNATIONAL ORTHOPEDIC CENTER FOR
   JOINT DISORDERS
David Schechter, M.D.
50 North LaCienega Boulevard, Suite 100
Beverly Hills, CA 90211
(310) 659-7414
Fax: (310) 659-3773
Web site: www.mindbodymedicine.com
Sports medicine specialist with a special
interest in mind-body approaches to pain

NATIONAL CHRONIC PAIN OUTREACH
   ASSOCIATION, INC.
7979 Old Georgetown Road, Suite 100
Bethesda, MD 20814-2429
(301) 652-4949
Fax: (301) 907-0745
An information clearinghouse; provides
referrals and publishes a newsletter.

NECK AND BACK PAIN ASSOCIATION
   OF AMERICA
2512 Mountain Road
Pasadena, MD 21122-0135
(410) 360-0014

AMERICAN CHRONIC PAIN ASSOCIATION
P.O. Box 850
Rocklin, CA 95677
(916) 632-0922
Web site: www.the.acpa.org
A self-help organization for pain patients
publishes a workbook and teaches coping
skills.

CLEVELAND CLINIC FOUNDATION
   RESEARCH INSTITUTE
9500 Euclid Avenue
Cleveland, OH 44195
(216) 444-2200
Web site: www.ccf.org

FOR THOSE IN PAIN, INC.
Bob Tellería, M.A.
P.O. Box 390845
Mountain View, CA 94039-0845
(650) 968-2323
Fax: (650) 968-2328
Web site: www.forthoseinpain.org
E-mail: fenix@best.com

JOHNS HOPKINS PAIN MANAGEMENT
   SERVICE
Baltimore, Maryland
(410) 955-8069

MAYO CLINIC'S PAIN MANAGEMENT
  CENTER
St. Mary's Hospital
Generes 2C
1216 2nd Street, SW
Rochester, MN 55902
(507) 255-5921

NEW YORK PAIN TREATMENT PROGRAM
30 East 40th Street, 11th Floor
New York, NY 10016
(212) 532-7999

PAIN CONTROL & REHABILITATION
  INSTITUTE
2786 North Decatur, Suite 220
Decatur, GA 30033
(404) 297-1400

ST. MARY'S SPINE CENTER
Connection-Spine Center
1 Shrader Street
San Francisco, CA 94117
(415) 750-5570

SETON SPINE CARE
1850 Sullivan Avenue, #200
Daly City, CA 94015
(415) 985-7500

UNIVERSITY OF WASHINGTON PAIN
  CENTER
4245 Roosevelt Way NE
Seattle, WA 98105
(206) 548-4282

Chapter 8

Medical Tests and Diagnostic Procedures

Philip Shtasel, D.O., F.A.O.C.R.
A Patient's Guide to Just What the Doctor Ordered. New York: Harper Perennial.

H. Winter Griffith, M.D. *The Complete Guide to Medical Tests.* Fishe Books.

Chapter 9

OFFICE OF CANCER COMMUNICATIONS
National Cancer Institute
Building 31, Room 10A03
9000 Rockville Pike
Bethesda, MD 20892-2580
(301) 496-5583
Web site: www.nci.nih.gov

AMERICAN CANCER SOCIETY (ACS)
1599 Clifton Road, N.E.
Atlanta, GA 30329
1-800-ACS-2345

NIH NEUROLOGICAL INSTITUTE
Bldg. 31, Room 8A16
31 Center Drive MSC 2540
Bethesda, MD 20892-2540
1-800-352-9424
Web site: www.ninds.nih.gov

THE NATIONAL CANCER INSTITUTE
HOTLINE
1-800-422-6237
The hotline personally disusses your specific questions and sends free brochures at your request.

Chapter 12

AMERICAN CHIROPRACTIC ASSOCIATION
1701 Clarendon Blvd.
Arlington, VA 22209
1-800-986-4636
Fax: (703) 243-2593
Web site: www.amerchiro.org

CONSORTIUM FOR CHIROPRACTIC
    RESEARCH
1095 Dunford Way
Sunnyvale, CA 94087

Michael Gazdar, D.C., C.C.S.P.
1776 Ygnacio Valley Road
Walnut Creek, CA 94598
(510) 939-BACK
Taking Your Back to the Future: How to Get a Painfree Back and Total Health with Chiropractic Care.
Web site: www.gazdar.com

THE NATIONAL COMMISSION FOR THE
    CERTIFICATION OF ACUPUNCTURISTS
11 Canal Center Plaza, Suite 300
Alexandria, VA 22314
(703) 548-9004
Fax: (703) 548-9079

PALMER COLLEGE OF CHIROPRACTIC WEST
90 E. Tasman Dr.
San Jose, CA 95134
(408) 944-6000
Web site: www.palmer.edu

Chapter 14

Mary Pullig Schatz, M.D. *Back Care Basics: A Doctors Gentle Yoga Program for Back and Neck Pain Relief.* Berkeley, Calif.: Rodmell Press, 1992.

YOGA TEACHER'S DIRECTORY
Find a yoga teacher with *Yoga Journal* magazine's directory of yoga teachers from around the country and the world. Updated each July.
For more information write to:
Yoga Jornal
2054 University Ave., #600
Berkeley, CA 94704
1-800-359-YOGA
(510) 841-9200
Web site: www.yogajournal.com

Richard Hittleman's Yoga, 28 Day Exercise Plan. New York: Workman Publishing Company, 1969.

Richard Hittleman's 30 Day Yoga Meditation Plan. Bantam Books, 1978.

Judith Lasater, Ph.D., P.T. *Relax and Renew: Restful Yoga for Stressful Times.* Rodmell Press, 1995.

Chapter 15

ACUPRESSURE INSTITUTE
1533 Shattuck Avenue
Berkeley, CA 94709
(510) 845-1059
1-800-442-2232 (Outside California)
Web site: www.acupressure.com
Also available on audiotape: *The Bum Back*

THE TRAGER® INSTITUTE
21 Locust
Mill Valley, CA 94941
(415) 388-2688
Fax: (415) 388-2710
E-mail: admin@trager.com

FELDENKRAIS® GUILD OF NORTH AMERICA
P.O. Box 11145
San Francisco, CA 94101
E-mail: feldngld@peak.org

FELDENKRAIS® CENTER FOR MOVEMENT
    EDUCATION
98 Cherry Street
San Francisco, CA 94131
(415) 826-3680

ALEXANDER TECHNIQUE CENTER
    OF WASHINGTON DC
Web site: www.alexandercenter.com

ALEXANDER TECHNIQUE
American Center for the Alexander
    Technique
142 West End Avenue
New York, NY 10023

HELLERWORK INTERNATIONAL
Karen Finan
Hellerwork™
(530) 926-2500

MENSENDIECK ENTERPRISES
P.O. Box 9450
Stanford, CA 94309
(650) 851-8184
Web site: www.backfitness.com

ASTON-PATTERNING
P.O. Box 3568
Incline Village, NV 89450
(702) 831-8228

PILATES
A Body of Work™
2797 Union Street
San Francisco, CA 94123
(415) 351-2797
Web site: www.abodyofwork.com

RAEL ISAACOWITZ
On Center Conditioning
441 N. Newport Blvd., Suite 203
Newport Beach, CA 92663

THE PHYSICAL MIND INSTITUTE
c/o Joan Breibart
1807 2nd Street, Suite 47
Santa Fe, NM 87505
(505) 988-1990
Web site: www.the-method.com

The Guild for Structural
   Integration
P.O. Box 1559
Boulder, CO 80306
(303) 447-0122
1-800-447-0150
Web site: www.rolfguild.org
E-mail: gsi@rolfguild.org

Tai Chi

Dahong Zhou, M.D. *The Chinese Exercise Book from Ancient to Modern China, Exercises for Well-Being and the Treatment of Illness.* Hartley & Marks, Ltd., 1994.

John "Shane" Watson with Mary Pritchaid, eds. *The Massage and Bodywork Resource Guide of North America.* Orenda Unity Press, 1983.

Chapter 16

Beverly Biondi
Back in Action Physical Therapy
P.O. Box 782
Sausalito, CA 94966
(415) 332-6061

Seton Spine Center
1850 Sullivan Avenue, #200
Daly City, CA 94015
(415) 985-7500

St. Mary's Medical Center-Health
   Connection-Spine Center
1 Shrader Street
San Francisco, CA 94117
(415) 750-5570
1-800-333-1355

Seton Spinecare
1850 Sullivan Avenue, #200
Daly City, CA 94015
(415) 985-7500
1-800-523-2225

Texas Back Institute
6300 West Parker Road
Plano, TX 75093
1-800-247-2225, press #1 for hotline
Web site: www.texasback.com

Health South Corporation
1 Health South Parkway
Birmingham, AL 35243
(205) 967-7116
Web site: www.healthsouth.com

Institute for Low Back and
   Neck Care
2800 Chicago Avenue South
Minneapolis, MN 55407-1382
(612) 879-2500

Institute for Spine Care
550 Harrison Street
Syracuse, NY 13202

Audiotape

David Schechter, M.D.
Get Rid of Back Pain, Basics of TMS and Treatment: Get on with Your Life
50 N. LaCienega Blvd., Suite 100
Beverly Hills, CA 90211
(310) 659-7414

A good Web site for general back questions and care: www.spine-dr.com

Chapter 22

BACK DESIGNS
1045 Ashby Avenue
Berkeley, CA 94710
Orders: 1-800-466-1341
Fax: (510) 549-0837
A good resource for ergonomics and
fielding questions.

BACK BE NIMBLE
(713) 521-0003
1-800-639-3746
Web site: www.backbenimble.com
On-line catalogue of self-care products,
orthopedic supplies, and travel-related
items for the back.

RELAX THE BACK FRANCHISING CO.
2101 Rosecrans Avenue, #1250
El Segundo, CA 90245
Web site: www.relaxtheback.com
The largest specialty retailer of back
products, a franchise with eighty stores
throughout the country.

THE HEALTHY BACK STORE
1201 University Avenue
San Diego, CA 92103
(619) 299-2225
1-800-469-2225
Web site: www.healthyback.com
Five retail stores throughout the country.
Call for extensive catalogue back
accoutrements.

GLOSSARY

Acupressure An ancient finger therapy for tension.

Acupuncture 3,000-year-old Chinese healing art that inserts fine needles into the body at specific points.

Alexander technique A type of bodywork that replaces dysfunctional body movements with functional ones by reteaching the body to move correctly.

Analgesics Painkillers.

Ankylosing spondylitis A chronic systemic inflammatory disorder of unknown cause.

Annulus fibrosis The outer part of a disk.

Aston-Patterning A type of bodywork that encourages body parts to cooperate with one another however they move.

Bak implants Large, hollow screws implanted inside the spine.

Benign tumor A tumor that limits growth to one area.

Bone scan A test where radioactive material is injected into the bloodstream. Used to detect bone fractures or infections.

Cartilage A fibrous connective tissue.

Cervical spine Pertaining to the neck.

Chi A vital energy running through your body.

Chondro sarcoma A type of bone cancer usually present in adults.

Chymopapain or chemonucleolysis An enzyme derived from the papaya fruit, which when injected into the nucleus of a herniated disk, shrinks the protruding area of the disk.

Computed axial tomography CAT uses a computer to generate X rays. The CAT scan shows soft tissue.

Diathermy A treatment to stimulate tissue under the skin.

Discogram A diagnostic test that aids in finding where the pain may be originating from. A dye is injected directly into the disk.

Electromyogram An invasive test that measures the speed of the motor nerve conduction with wires inserted into the muscles and nerves.

Ewing's sarcoma A type of bone cancer.

Facet joints The gliding joints between the vertebrae that guide, direct, and limit the movement of the spine.

Feldenkrais A type of bodywork called functional integration, it teaches one to learn to move in a graceful way.

Fibromyalgia A syndrome characterized by chronic musculoskeletal pain throughout the body.

Foramenotomy A surgical procedure that provides a passageway for the spinal nerves from spinal stenosis.

Fusion A surgical procedure used to stabilize vertebrae, where bones are bridged together.

General practitioner A family doctor or internist.

Hellerwork A type of bodywork that uses some deep-tissue manipulation, verbal interaction, and a focus on individual personality traits.

Herniated disk A protrusion of the nucleus pulposus, causing the center to bulge or seep out.

Idiopathic Of unknown etiology or origin.

Juvenile kyphosis Another name for vertebral osteochondritis.

Kyphosis An abnormal condition of the vertebral column.

Kyphotic curve A convex or rounded curvature of the thoracic spine.

Laminectomy A surgical posterior removal of a portion of the disk.

Laser arthroscopic microdiscectomy A minimally noninvasive back surgery using an arthroscope and laser fiber.

Leg discrepancy A difference in length between legs.

Ligaments Bands of fibrous tissue that connect bone and cartilage.

Lordosis Swayback, or an exaggeration of the normal lumbar curve.

Lordotic curve A concave curvature of the spine.

Lumbago Chronic pain in the lumbar area.

Lumbar spine The lower back area.

Magnetic resonance imagining A test that uses a magnetic force with a computer to view the body. MRI shows soft tissue, nerves, and bones.

Malignant tumor A tumor that metastasizes or grows elsewhere in your body.

Meningitis An inflammation of the tissues that cover the brain and spinal cord.

Meningoioms Benign tumors in the thoracic spine.

Mensendieck A type of bodywork that corrects body mechanics, muscle function, and posture.

Meridians Invisible pathways in Chinese medicine.

Microdiscectomy A surgical procedure using a microscope and a small incision. Not considered a percutaneous procedure.

Minimally noninvasive procedure A surgical procedure that uses an arthroscope or endoscope. No incision or stitching is involved.

Multiple myeloma A cancer that affects white blood cells.

Muscles Providers of strength and movement for the body.

Myelogram A diagnostic test in which a dye is injected into the spinal canal. The test gives information about the nerves, disk, and bones.

Neurologist A doctor who specializes in neurological or nerve disorders.

NSAIDs Nonsteroidal anti-inflammatory drugs.

Nucleus pulposus The jellylike center of the disk.

Orthopedist A doctor who specializes in bone, joints, and muscle disorders.

Osteoarthritis A noninflammatory degenerative joint disease chiefly occurring in older persons. Also called degenerative arthritis.

Osteomyelitis An infection from the bloodstream that has reached the spinal area.

Osteopath A doctor of osteopathy.

Osteopathy A system of medicine that emphasizes normal body mechanics and manipulative methods of detecting and correcting faulty structure.

Osteoporosis A condition that weakens the bones due to loss in bone strength.

Osteosarcoma A type of bone cancer.

Pedicle screws Used to stabilize the spine after spinal injury or to correct other abnormalities.

Percutaneous laser discectomy A minimally noninvasive surgery that uses laser energy.

Percutaneous spine surgical procedures The latest in spine surgery. The procedure goes under the skin without cutting or stitching.

Physiatrist A doctor who specializes in musculoskeletal rehabilitation.

Physical therapist A back educator who teaches therapies for your back.

Pilates A form of classic exercise that works with a form of resistance control to teach the individual to work from the inside out.

Piriformis syndrome A condition whereby the piriformis muscle entraps the sciatic nerve.

Polymyalgia rheumatica An episodic inflammatory disease of the large arteries.

Reflexology A Western pressure-point therapy that focuses on the feet.

Reiter's syndrome A group of symptoms of unknown etiology compromising urethritis, conjunctivitis, and arthritis chiefly afflicting men.

Rheumatoid arthritis A form of arthritis.

Rolfing A type of bodywork called structural integration where deep manipulation of the connective tissue occurs.

Sacrum The triangle bone just below the lumbar vertebrae.

Scheuerman's disease Another name for vertebral osteochondritis.

Sciatica A syndrome characterized by pain radiating from the back into the buttocks and into the lower extremities, caused by a ruptured disk impinging on the nerve root.

Scoliosis A lateral curve of the spine, specifically the upper spine.

Shiatsu A method of finger pressure used in Japan.

Spina bifida The failure of an infants spine to close prior to birth.

Spinal stenosis A degenerative process of the narrowing of the spinal canal.

Spondylolisthesis The sliding forward of the entire vertebral body due to ligament and muscle weakness.

Spondylolysis A stress fracture that develops in the pars interarticularis of one or more of the vertebrae.

Stabilization Impeccable spinal body mechanics.

Subluxation A problem that exists when a joint does not function properly.

Tai chi A form of exercise or martial art originating in China to reduce stress and enhance health.

Thoracic spine The middle back or area between the the chest and pelvis.

Trager A type of bodywork known as psychophysical integration that uses simple movements to enhance body flexibility.

Transcutaneous electrical nerve stimulation An electrode stimulation to help reduce pain.

Ultrasound A treatment to stimulate tissue under the skin by generating heat.

Vertebra Any of the thirty-three bones of the spinal column.

Vertebral osteochondritis Inflammation of both bone and cartilage.

Whiplash A term applied to injury of the spine and spinal cord occurring as the result of a rapid acceleration or deceleration of the body.

X ray A test that shows bone, but not soft tissue.

Yoga A series of postures or poses that enhance musculoskeletal strength, flexibility, and balance.

BIBLIOGRAPHY

Abraham, Edward A., M.D. *Freedom From Back Pain, An Orthopedist's Self-Help Guide.* Emmaus, Pa.: Rodale Press, 1986.

The Back Almanac. Oakland, Calif.: Lanier Publishing International, Ltd., 1992.

Bone Cancer & Research Report. Bethesda, Md.: National Cancer Institute, 1990.

Bonnick, Sydney Lou, M.D., F.A.C.P. *The Osteoporosis Handbook, Every Woman's Guide to Prevention and Treatment.* Dallas, Tex.: Taylor Publishing Company, 1994.

Brewer, Earl J., Jr., M.D. and Kathy Cochran Angel. *The Arthritis Sourcebook.* Los Angeles: Lowell House, 1993.

Cailliet, Rene, M.D. *Neck and Arm Pain.* Philadelphia: F.A. Davis Company, 1991.

————. *Low Back Pain Syndrome*, 4th ed. Philadelphia: F.A. Davis Company, 1988.

Catalano, Ellen Mohr, M.A. *The Chronic Pain Control Workbook, A Step-by-Step Guide for Coping With and Overcoming Your Pain.* Oakland, Calif.: New Harbinger Publications, Inc., 1987.

Davidson, Paul, M.D. *Chronic Muscle Pain Syndrome.* New York: Berkeley Books, 1988.

Faye, Leonard. *Good Bye Back Pain.* Los Angeles: Weaver Publishing, 1990.

Fine, Judylaine. *Conquering Back Pain, A Comprehensive Guide.* New York: Prentice Hall, 1985.

Fraser, Richard, M.D. and Ann Forer. *The Well Informed Patient's Guide to Back Surgery.* New York: Dell Publishing, 1992.

Griffith, H. Winter, M.D. *The Complete Guide to Prescription & Non-Prescription Drugs.* New York: The Body Press, 1988.

————. *The Complete Guide to Medical Tests.* Tucson, Ariz.: Fishe Books, 1988.

Haldeman, Scott, D.C., M.D., Ph.D., David Chapman Smith, L.L.B., and Donald M. Petersen, Jr. *Guidelines for Chiropractic Quality Assurance and Practice Parameters.* Gaithersburg, Md.: Aspen Publication,1993.

Hochschuler, Stephen, M.D. *Back In Shape, A Back Owner's Maual,* Boston: Houghton Mifflin, 1991.

Hochsuler, Stephen, M.D., Howard B. Cotler, M.D., and Richard D. Guyer, M.D. *Rehabilitation of the Spine.* St. Louis, Mo.: Science and Practice, Mosby, 1993.

Journal of Musculoskeletal Medicine. January 1992.

Hope Through Research: National Institute of Neurological Disorders and Strokes. Bethesda, Md.: National Institutes of Health, 1993.

Klein, Arthur C. and Dava Sobel. *Backache Relief.* New York: NAL Books, 1985.

Long, James W., M.D. and James J. Rybacki, Pharm.D. *The Essential Guide To Prescription Drugs-Everything You Need to Know for Safe Drug Use.* New York: Harper Perennial, 1994.

McKenzie, Robin, F.N.Z.S.P., DIP, M.T. *Treat Your Own Back.* New Zealand: Spinal Publications Ltd., 1985.

Mosby's Medical and Nursing Dictionary, 2d ed. St. Louis, Mo.: The C.V. Mosby Company, 1986.

Potash, Warren J., et al., *Your Lower Back.* Jenkintown, Pa.: Paragon Communications, Inc., 1993.

Renfro, Mary, Chloe Fisher, and Suzanne Arms. *Bestfeeding: Getting Breastfeeding Right for You.* Berkeley, Calif.: Celestial Arts, 1990.

Sarno, John E., M.D. *Healing Back Pain, The Mind-Body Connection.* New York: Warner Books, Inc., 1991.

Schatz, Mary Pullig, M.D. *Back Care Basics, A Doctor's Gentle Yoga Program for Back and Neck Relief.* Berkeley, Calif.: Rodmell Press, 1992.

Sherman, James R. *How to Overcome a Bad Back.* Pathway Books, 1980.

Simons, Anne, M.D., Bobbie Hasselbring, and Michael Castleman. *Before You Call the Doctor: Safe Effective Self-Care for Over 300 Common Medical Problems.* New York: Fawcett Columbine, 1992.

Sobel, David S. and Tom Ferguson. *The People's Book of Medical Tests.* New York: Summit, 1985.

Sternback. Richard A. *Mastering Pain, A Twelve-Step Program for Coping With Chronic Pain.* New York: Ballantine Books, 1987.

Tarlov, Edward, M.D., and David D'Costa. *Back Attack.* Boston-Toronto: Little Brown and Company, 1985

White, Arthur H., M.D. *Back School and Other Conservative Approaches to Low Back Pain.* St. Louis, Mo.: Mosby, 1983.

White, Arthur H., M.D., and Robert Anderson. *Conservative Care of Low Back Pain.* Williams & Wilkins, 1991.

White, Augustus A., III, M.D. *Your Aching Back, A Doctor's Guide to Relief.* New York: Simon & Shuster: Fireside Books, 1990.

White, Lynne A. *Spine State-of-the-Art Reviews.* Philadelphia: Hanley & Belfus, Inc., 1991.

The Womanly Art of Breastfeeding. Franklin Park, Ill.: La Leche League International, 1991.

Zimmerman, Julie, P.T. *Chronic Back Pain: Moving On.* Brunswick, Maine: Biddle Publishing Co., 1991.

———. *The Almanac of Back Pain Treatments*. Brunswick, Maine: Biddle Publishing Co., 1991.

INDEX